THE CHALLENGE OF MEDICALLY UNEXPLAINED DISORDERS (M.U.D.)

By

C. Philip O'Carroll, MD

TABLE OF CONTENTS

Introduction

Several years ago, Dr. Matthew Burke from the Neurology Department at Beth Israel Deaconess Medical Center wrote a brief article titled *"It's All in Your Head – Medicine's Silent Epidemic."* He referred to the multiple "functional disorders" confronting neurologists, including fibromyalgia, chronic fatigue syndrome, brain fog, and many others. He called it a silent epidemic because there are no metrics available to estimate the scope of the problem. As he wrote, "The magnitude of the crisis is difficult to demonstrate because these patients largely elude the billing codes used for case ascertainment in large population-based studies." He argued that to address this epidemic, we must first change the medical culture.

But before we can address this epidemic, we must first estimate its scope! To quote Lord Kelvin, "When you can measure what you are speaking about and express it in numbers, you know something about it… When you cannot express it in numbers, your knowledge is of a meager and unsatisfactory kind."

This is not just an academic issue. We have the most expensive healthcare system in the world, yet we also have the lowest satisfaction ratings compared to other developed countries. It's likely that billions of dollars are wasted each year in the hunt for classifiable diseases when, in fact, the symptoms stem from behavioral or stress-related issues in patients' lives. It is estimated that up to two-thirds of patients presenting to primary care have no identifiable or classifiable diseases, and the incidence is even higher in specialty care. These disorders range from conditions with no obvious pathology, such as fibromyalgia and chronic fatigue, to more common ailments like headache, back pain, and gastrointestinal disorders, which have become chronic and resistant to treatment. Chronic pain is a prominent feature in many of these cases.

The psychological and medical disciplines view these disorders through their own biases. Doctors tend to adhere to the medical model, often spending lavishly on tests and treatments in search of disease, while psychological practitioners view "unease" through a bewildering variety of overlapping diagnostic labels.

Medical training, the "medical model," is exclusively focused on disease, with an emphasis on the more unusual and exotic conditions, the "fascinoma" — a rare condition that may never be encountered in clinical practice.

This approach was best exemplified by the brain-cutting conference held every Thursday at Mass General Hospital. A case was presented by a resident in training, followed by x-rays and scans, a learned dissertation, and differential diagnoses. The moment of truth came when the brain of the deceased patient was presented on a marble platter, and the neuropathologist made the first slice with a pearl-handled blade. A frisson of anticipation rippled through the audience as we waited for the revelation. There was an underlying assumption, never questioned, that there would be obvious pathology. No pathology, no brain-cutting conference. It's certain that functional disorders did not feature prominently at this venue.

The issue with rare diseases is that they are rare! More often than not, the doctor, whether in primary or specialty care, is confronted with everyday problems like pain, fatigue, insomnia, and gut disorders. Chronic pain is the most frequent of these. For the neurologist, chronic headache is common, as are other puzzling disorders like brain fog, chronic fatigue, and fibromyalgia. These disorders do not feature in our training; they don't conform to the medical model. It took many years to understand and respect these amorphous symptoms and to realize that they were also real and "organic," just not conforming to the accepted definition of organicity.

We are products of a medical system that assumes every patient we see has a recognizable, classifiable disease. Clearly, this is not the case. Yet there are no guidelines for how to deal with non-diseases. Some attempts have been made to develop a "mind-body" approach, but these often devolve into neuromythology. Patients are increasingly turning to internet "shamans" and "Dr. Google" because medicine ignores two-thirds of the patient population. We need a new approach to address this silent epidemic. The traditional medical model has served us well, but it urgently needs an overhaul if it is to meet the needs of modern humans.

NOTE:

This is not a serious academic treatise with lengthy references and citations. Literature on medically unexplained conditions is often confusing and contradictory. It's easy to get lost in the underbrush of taxonomy, which largely falls under the domain of the psychiatric profession. I have included only the most relevant sources on which I have personally relied. For the enthusiast, feel free to enter the nomenclature thicket — but you may never emerge! It's a short book; most books would benefit from brevity, especially academic tomes. When King George III was presented with the third volume of Edward Gibbon's massive six-volume work, *The History of the Decline and Fall of the Roman Empire*, he supposedly remarked, "Another damned fat book! Always scribble, scribble, scribble, eh, Mr. Gibbon?" (No apologies for the frequent literary, philosophical, and theological allusions; I grew up without cell phones or television or the damnable curse of social media.)

I believe it's important to understand the evolution of our thinking as physicians, so I have included a brief chapter on the history of the medical model. I am to be forgiven for waxing philosophical occasionally, especially on the mind-body problem, since that is the dilemma patients and doctors must deal with on a daily basis, even if they don't realize it. I have also devoted several chapters to basic neuroscience, particularly the neuroscience of stress, as it is difficult to fully grasp the impact of life stress without some understanding of basic anatomy. As a practicing physician with over 50 years of struggling to understand human beings, I've gathered anecdotes and insights, hoarding them like a squirrel collecting acorns. Unfortunately, I've long since forgotten their source. Apologies if I fail in attribution.

I am a clinician, a neurologist, seeing patients who present with both disease and "unease," and I am painfully aware that I lack the resources to treat the latter. There is no new, all-encompassing medical model on the horizon that can embrace the full spectrum of human suffering. Still, I am encouraged by the words of William James: "A large acquaintance with particulars makes us wiser than the possession of abstract formulas, however deep."

This is what we physicians have — particulars, called patients.

(JAMA Neurology Dec. 2019, Vol. 76, 12)

Chapter 1

The Medical Model, Past and Present

Entering the world of the MUDs is to enter a murky, uncertain terrain with few guideposts. Doctors love disorders that conform to the "medical model," clear-cut and unambiguous. If that's what a budding physician is seeking, I would advise they consider veterinary medicine or orthopedic surgery, where the pathology is stark and visible.

Much is written about the so-called medical model, either praising it or pointing out its limitations. A model is a framework, a way of thinking, a theoretical basis for understanding and explaining real-world systems. Thomas Kuhn, the eminent philosopher of science, popularized the term "paradigm." He wrote that paradigms or models can be very useful in understanding complex structures, but they all suffer from a common malady, which he called "paradigm paralysis" (by now a much-hackneyed term). Simply put, paradigms or models adhere to principles that are rarely expressed, accepted as universal truths, and resistant to change. In this, the medical model is not unique. There is an oft-told anecdote concerning Lord Kelvin, the father of atomic theory.

In an address to the British Association for the Advancement of Science in 1900, he stated, "There is nothing new to be discovered in physics now; all that remains is more and more precise measurements." Five years later, a lowly, underpaid level three clerk in a Swiss patent office named Albert Einstein, published his paper on Special Relativity and shattered Lord Kelvin's worldview. Einstein's model did not negate the physics of Isaac Newton. Stand in front of a speeding bus, and you will find that Newtonian physics is still applicable. Einstein's model merely showed that in certain circumstances, Newton's physics did not apply. Lord Kelvin, in another example of paradigm paralysis, famously questioned the utility of wireless transmission, saying, "Wireless telegraphy is all very well, but I'd rather send a message by a boy on a pony."

Years later, Einstein himself became a victim of another paradigm shift with the development of quantum mechanics. According to this model, what happens at the ultramicroscopic level is completely different from what happens at the macro level. The idea that two particles, continents apart, are somehow entangled and have the capacity to influence each other's properties was dismissed as "spooky science" by Einstein. He could not accept the apparent chaos and unpredictability implied by the quantum model and fought against it for the rest of his life. Somewhat peevishly, he complained, "God does not play dice with the universe."

Ancient

The medical model has evolved over many thousands of years. Long before science, there was religion. Religion offered a coherent narrative for human misery, suffering, and death. It provided simple answers to eternal questions: "Why am I here? Why do I suffer? Why do I die?" The answer was straightforward: we are sinful creatures, expelled from paradise by an angry God. Our sin? We were too curious; we succumbed to the serpent's wiles and were banished from Eden. Pain, suffering, and death are the price we pay for our disobedience. (I wonder if our sin was indeed so great that it required an all-powerful God to torture and kill his own son!)

The word pain is derived from the Latin *poena*, meaning punishment. In this system, the priest or shaman was the instrument of healing, interceding with the gods on our behalf. In many cultures, they remain a powerful force. A good physician should have a little shaman; our patients still attribute magical qualities to their doctor.

Medical science slowly emerged in the West, with the towering figure of Hippocrates (460 BC–375 BC) and his humoral theory. This theory dominated Western medicine for thousands of years. According to this model, there are four distinct bodily fluids or "humors" in a person: black bile, yellow bile, blood, and phlegm.

It is the balance of these humors that defines good health. An excess or deficiency of these humors could lead to various conditions. For instance, an excess of black bile could lead to melancholy (Greek: *melas* = black, *chole* = bile). (There are still echoes of humoral theory in modern psychopharmacology; ancient healers balanced the humors, while modern psychiatrists balance neurotransmitters.)

The humoral theory was universally accepted by physicians up until the mid-19th century. For thousands of years, medical training consisted of memorizing the works of ancient healers, especially Galen (129 AD–216 AD). His views, based on balancing the humors, dominated Western medical science for more than 1,300 years. The flaw at the heart of Galen's model was his ignorance of anatomy and physiology. The Judeo-Christian taboo against dissecting the human body meant there was no real medical science. As a result, Galen's study of the human body was limited to chance encounters and the occasional observation of wounded gladiators or soldiers. Little by little, respect for Galen's authority gave way to the need to "see-to-know," and the return of cadaver dissection. Remarkably, Galen's teachings served as the guiding force in science and medicine for over 1,300 years. Small wonder that the medical profession was often the subject of sarcasm and ridicule. "The best doctor is one you run into in an emergency but cannot find". (Molière, *The Doctor in Spite of Himself*)

Medieval

The scientific model truly began with Vesalius (Andreas Witting 1514–1564). He opened the human body to dissection and revealed disease to be a localized, discernible problem in the body, not an affliction from the gods or an imbalance in the humors. His great work, *De Humani Corporis Fabrica* (1543), "On the Workings of the Human Body," is considered one of the most important books in medical science. His dissection of the brain was remarkable in its accuracy; however, he was mystified as to how the brain could give rise to the mind. He wrote, "I can, to some degree, follow the brain's functions in dissections of living animals, with sufficient probability and truth, but I am unable to understand how the brain can perform its functions of imagining, meditating, thinking, and remembering." We haven't made much progress solving that riddle. In fact, if he were resurrected today, he would still be mystified as to how a lump of soggy grey matter produces consciousness and mind.

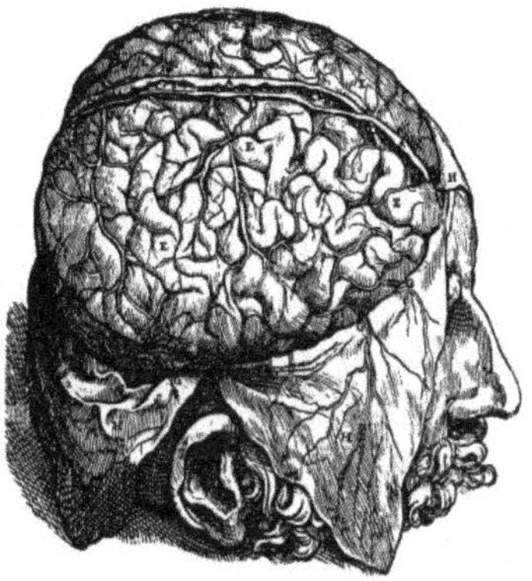

FIGURE 1: DE HUMANI CORPORIS FABRICA (1543)

Predictably, his great work met with resistance from those entrenched in the ancient model. He was investigated by the Spanish Inquisition for violating the taboo of human dissection, but before they could inflict any of their dreaded punishments, he went on a pilgrimage to Jerusalem and died en route. (One might wonder what penance would have been levied on William Harvey, the discoverer of the circulation of the blood. He was working at a time when fresh, dead bodies were hard to come by, so he dissected his own father and sister!)

Modern

Only in the mid-19th century did truly scientific medicine emerge, with the rise of the Viennese school of medicine under the leadership of Rudolf Virchow (1821-1902). He is often referred to as the "undertaker" because he buried the medieval concepts of disease. Ironically, he also buried the concept of holism, which was the basis of ancient medicine. (The word holism is derived from the Greek word *holos,* whole). We have been trying to regain it ever since. His publication in 1855 of his monumental work *Cellular Pathology as Based Upon Physiological and Pathological Histology* laid out the fundamental principles and cornerstone of our current model. He stated: "There are no diseases but diseases of cells and organs." This is the "mission statement," the ultimate expression of our biomechanical, reductionistic model that reduces the patient to a body to be intervened upon rather than a person to be cared for. In this way of thinking, the only diseases were those that could be observed and proven. The myriads of medically unexplained disorders could not be classified so easily and were largely ignored. They still are!

The medical model has served us well, liberating medicine from superstition and quackery, but it now desperately needs a "paradigm shift." It is still mired in 19th-century thought. It is strictly reductionist, ignoring the contribution of the mind/brain. It is a disease model, but there is even no consensus as to what constitutes a disease. Cancer and tuberculosis can be classified as real diseases, but what about alcoholism, drug addiction, or attention deficit disorder? Tuberculosis can be considered a real disease, but the incidence of TB began to decline long before antibiotics, due to social and economic factors. Doctors often take undue credit for the achievements of engineers and public health workers. The combined death rate from scarlet fever, diphtheria, whooping cough, and measles among children up to age 15 shows that nearly 90% of the total decline in mortality between 1860 and 1965 had occurred before the introduction of antibiotics and widespread immunization.

With the emergence of the psychological disciplines, the concept of disease has become even more confounding, with new "diseases" arriving and disappearing with every new edition of the DSM, the Diagnostic and Statistical Manual, the bible of psychiatry. The American Psychiatric Association (APA) proclaims new diseases and abolishes old ones, not by science but by consensus. There just isn't enough science!

The current medical system works well with classifiable diseases but struggles with the myriad of disorders that defy neat categorization—the medically unexplained disorders. Ignoring this huge population of patients is no longer acceptable.

(T. Kuhn. The Structure of Scientific Revolution. 2nd Edition. University of Chicago Press. 1970.
Ivan Illich. Limits To Medicine M and S. 1976. C. Smuts. Holism and Evolution. N.Y. Macmillan. 1926)

Chapter 2

The Confusing, Bewildering World of the Medically Unexplained Disorders

"It is devilish to suffer from a pain but is all but nameless. Blessed are they that are stricken with identifiable, classifiable diseases, for at least other people know what is the matter with them and will listen to their bellyaching with sympathy." — George Orwell

John was an 18-year-old boy who sought my help for relentless, chronic daily headaches. The disorder began about nine months earlier. He described the pain as "24/7," which never varied in intensity or location. "It's not pain; it's tightness, a pressure in my head," he said, but it still felt like a "10 out of 10." Before the headaches began, he was a high-achieving student. However, since the onset of his condition, his grades dropped, and his parents had to homeschool him. Yet, there was no improvement in his pain or grades.

During his initial visit, John sat quietly, allowing his father to speak. His father, an engineer, with an engineer's logic, felt that something was wrong with John that was "being missed," despite multiple MRI scans, two spinal taps, and blood tests. His father suggested it could be "autoimmune." I realized that conventional questioning wasn't going to help, so I asked why John's mother was not present. Father responded without emotion, "She's dying". I learned John's mother, a Chinese native, had been diagnosed with a type of stomach cancer that's common in China, and invariably fatal. She was 48 years old. John's symptoms started shortly after his mother's diagnosis. At the mention of his mother's impending death, John looked distraught. I walked him to the psychologist's office next to mine, a therapist who had been a part of the clinic for many years. After several sessions, John's head pain and pressure disappeared.

That was almost ten years ago. John is now pursuing his Ph.D. at MIT and visits me occasionally when he comes with his father, who has developed Parkinson's disease. Several times, I've asked him, "Did you grasp the connection between your head pain and your mother's diagnosis?" His answer is always the same: "I'm sorry, doctor, I just don't get it." After 50 years as a physician, I still marvel at the firewall between bodily symptoms and feelings. I'm equally baffled by the failure of physicians to ask personal questions like, WHERE IS MOM?

One day, we will all die from a classifiable disease unless we fall victim to trauma or another mishap. But over the course of our lives, we are more likely to suffer from ailments that don't fit into any convenient medical category. The body is always complaining, whether it's a sniffle, a stiff neck, that nagging back pain, or an upset stomach. We endure these aches and pains with over-the-counter remedies, most of which are ineffective. Yet, occasionally, these symptoms cross a threshold, prompting a visit to the doctor (but only after consulting Dr. Google), resulting in several fatal "diagnoses." A wise physician will listen and reassure, and often that is the cure.

In his 1911 play, The Doctor's Dilemma, George Bernard Shaw describes Dr. Sir Ralph Bloomfield Bonington as follows: "Cheering, reassuring, healing by the mere incompatibility of disease or anxiety with his welcome presence. Even broken bones, it is said, have been known to unite at the sound of his voice".

These days, Dr. Sir Ralph would be too busy inputting data into the electronic health record to even look at his patient.

But there is another presentation that physicians face daily, no longer the predictable short-lived symptoms that are merely a reflection of everyday life stress. These are the medically unexplained disorders — no longer transient, but chronic and resistant to treatment.

They go by many names, reflecting our own lack of clarity. For the MD, they are functional, psychosomatic, psychological, central sensitivity disorders, but most appropriately, *medically unexplained disorders* (MUDs). With the rise of psychological disciplines, there are even more labels, somatoform, somatization disorders, conversion disorders, and, of course, hysteria. (Yes, it still exists. It was declared dead and removed from the DSM-III in 1980, but it persists in the DSM-V as *functional neurological disorder* or *conversion disorder*). Whatever the label, it's here that we encounter heightened psychological distress, childhood abuse, PTSD, depression, and anxiety.

Arthur Barsky, a professor of psychiatry at Harvard, has researched this "no-man's-land" between mind and body medicine for decades. His label, *functional somatic syndromes*, at least implies a disturbance in bodily function if not anatomy. He writes, "Functional somatic syndromes are determined by multiple factors and are as much shaped by psychological, sociocultural, and circumstantial forces, so they resist localization anywhere within our medical or psychiatric taxonomy." Unfortunately, employing a definition that resists localization of these symptoms means they also resist measurement.

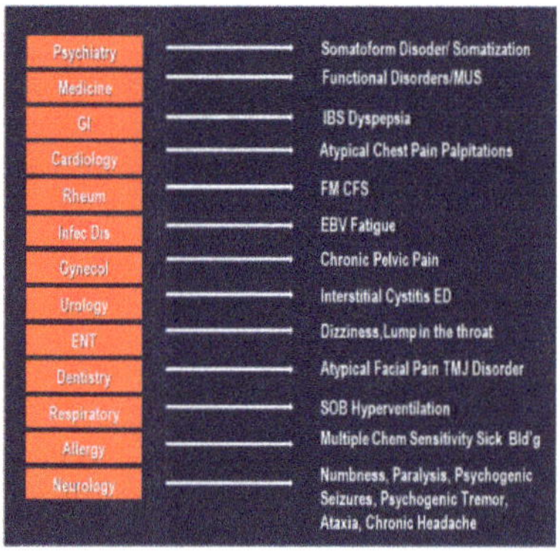

Every specialty has its own distinctive MUD. The gastroenterologist has irritable bowel syndrome (IBS), the cardiologist has palpitations and atypical chest pain, the rheumatologist is burdened with fibromyalgia and chronic fatigue, the infectious disease specialist deals with Epstein-Barr and Chronic Lyme, the gynecologist addresses chronic pelvic pain, the urologist faces irritable bladder syndrome, and the dentist treats TMJ. But the neurologist claims the top billing. We see numbness, paralysis, bizarre movement disorders, and non-epileptiform seizures (formerly called pseudo-seizures, as they are identical to real seizures, except for a normal EEG). These neurological symptoms are unique enough to warrant their own category, *functional neurological disorders* (FNDs).

Our medical model is ill-equipped to deal with these disorders. Doctors are trained in a biomechanical model of disease that treats organs, not people. Consequently, as the familiar adage goes, when the only tool you have is a hammer, every problem looks like a nail. We have difficulty coping with symptoms that don't fit into a neat category, that are chronic and often encrusted with multiple layers, behavioral, psychological, and social. The poet W. H. Auden, himself a chronic headache sufferer, wrote, "Under the look of fatigue, behind the migraine and the sigh, there is always another story. There is more than meets the eye." Much of the time, the "more" in question is stress and anxiety, the scourge of modern humans.

Chronic stress has been called "The Black Death" of the 21st century. The stress may be current and more easily identified by the patient when explored, or it may stem from the past in the form of unresolved or unprocessed trauma. In either case, this stress often becomes a central underlying feature of many of these disorders. It is estimated that 50–70% of primary care visits are ultimately traceable to conditions related to or exacerbated by stress, and that percentage is even higher in specialty or secondary care settings.

Within medical practice, this group of patients is often disparaged and labeled as "crocks, neurotics, and hysterics." They are frequently met with condescension and dismissal, leading them to seek help from alternative healers, who are more than willing to offer diagnoses and treatments. These healers fill the void created by our inability to understand and treat these disorders. These patients live in the shadowlands of medicine; it is time to reclaim them with understanding and empathy.

I am not merely suggesting handholding or commiseration. It is essential to emphasize that these symptoms are organic and real, but our concept of "organic" needs to evolve. We must recognize the role of both the brain and mind in these disorders. Stress, whether current or past, affects brain structure and function. Understanding and explaining the brain-body connection can be a powerful, validating force. It's not "all in your mind", it's all in your brain. Psychology is Biology. I realize this is a form of reductionism, but it's a more acceptable one. Patients are not philosophers; they simply want reassurance that their symptoms are real.

There are multiple on-ramps to the bewildering world of MUDs and PUDs (Psychiatrically Unexplained Disorders), but there is a fundamental mechanism underlying them all, the conversion of the mental into the physical, the psyche into soma.

McFarlane, A.: The Conundrum of Medically Unexplained Symptoms – Questions to Consider, *Psychosomatics 49:5. Sept. – Oct. 2008*)
Barsky, AJ: Functional Somatic Syndromes. *Amer. Int. Med. 1999*
Kroenke, K.: J. Clin. Psychiatry. 1998. *59, (Supp 20) 5-8*
Moss-Morris: To Lump or To Split. *Psychosomatic Medicine 68: 463-469. 2006*
Per Fink: One Single Diagnosis, Bodily Distress Syndrome. J. Psychosomatic Research 68. (2010) 415-416
Dimsdale, J: Somatoform Disorders *Psychosomatics 2011, '52: 154-9*

Chapter 3

Characteristics of M.U.D.s

These poorly understood conditions do not follow the medical model. They are mysterious and ever-changing. In this day and age, social media plays a major role in their appearance and disappearance, often with disorienting speed. Whatever the label, they share very similar characteristics:

Common Clinical Presentation ("Facts") of MUDs

- They involve multiple symptoms but lack objective signs or identifiable biomarkers,
- There is often a history of depression and anxiety, along with a family history of these disorders,
- A history of childhood abuse or neglect is frequently present,
- Pain is a prominent feature in many of these conditions in the modern era,
- There may be a growing skepticism toward institutions and traditional expertise, with many patients turning to alternative sources of information and personal research,
- Patients often take an active role in understanding and framing their symptoms, sometimes adopting medical language and frameworks that resonate with their experience,
- Self-help and advocacy communities are widespread and can provide validation and support, while also shaping how these conditions are understood,
- Pharmaceutical approaches may reinforce a disease-based model, particularly when treatment options are available,

- Psychological explanations are sometimes experienced by patients as dismissive rather than helpful, leading to understandable resistance or frustration,
- Females outnumber males in nearly every category of medically unexplained illness.

Some doctors try to help, but others exploit the vulnerability of sufferers, charging vast sums for unproven remedies. Beware of "wellness" and "integrative" clinics. Many rely on pseudoscience and salesmanship to sell their expensive treatments. The more time, hope and resources patients invest into this type of "treatment", the more they are motivated to believe in its potential power to heal them.

"Lumpers Vs Splitters"

These disorders do not fit easily into one category. There is an ongoing debate between lumpers and splitters: is there only one disorder with different manifestations or multiple distinct conditions? I am a splitter. Psychiatrists and psychologists tend to see patients with behavioral or psychological symptoms, often with no obvious structural basis, but the medical doctor sees another type of MUD. These are disorders that start with a well-defined pathological basis but transition into the medically mysterious category as they become chronic. These are the conditions doctors face daily, disorders that begin with clear pathology but transform over time to enter the realm of medically unexplained disorders. The term chronic is always associated with these conditions, meaning long-lasting, and pain features prominently.

Nonfatal diseases are chronic by definition, providing ample time for behavioral and psychological factors to "hijack" the original pathology. The longer the disorder lasts, the more difficult it is to disentangle the contribution of individual factors. Headache, back pain, or gut conditions are no great mystery, but for various reasons, they may become chronic and resistant to treatment. Dissociated from their pathophysiologic origins, they drift into MUD territory. There are different transformative factors at work, not always behavioral. These disorders have their own niche in the MUD landscape and should not be "lumped" with the more nebulous disorders that have no obvious pathological basis.

Pain features prominently in many medically unexplained disorders. Paul Briquet, 1796-1881, one of the prominent writers on hysteria, wrote, "Pain in the muscles is so common with this neurosis that it is rare not to have muscle pain during the course of the illness." (Traite de l'hysterie, 1859). A heightened sensitivity to painful and even nonpainful stimuli is a feature of irritable bowel syndrome (IBS), low back pain, fibromyalgia (FM), interstitial cystitis (IC), and pelvic pain. The term "central sensitivity disorder" is appropriate, as it emphasizes altered central processing in the brain rather than peripheral pathology. The "target organ" may vary, but the alteration in brain circuitry is the underlying pathology, often the result of unrelenting and severe stress, especially in childhood.

The neurologist often encounters a different form of medically unexplained disorders, and they are unique enough to warrant their own label: Functional Neurologic Disorders (FNDs). Patients may present with psychogenic non-epileptiform seizures (PNES), paralysis, bizarre movement disorders, and non-physiologic sensory disorders. To add to the confusion, these disorders have been labeled as "conversion disorder". If they see the neurologist, it is a functional neurologic disorder; if they see the psychiatrist, then it is a conversion disorder. (It is reminiscent of Aesop's fable about the blind men confronted with an elephant. Each one describes a single feature of the animal without grasping the whole.)

Regardless of the manifestations or labels, these disorders represent the conversion of mind into matter, the mental into the physical. Different brain circuits are recruited in the varied presentations, but the underlying mechanism remains the same: emotions and mental experiences are converted into physical form.

(Some would argue that the term Functional Neurologic Disorder should be an all-embracing label for all these disorders since they all emanate from the brain. However, the term Functional Neurologic Disorder should probably be reserved for those with a "neurological" presentation.)

Fink, P. (2015). Medically Unexplained Symptoms: Definitions and Diagnostic Approaches. LANCET PSYCHIATRY.
Katon, W. (2003) Clinical Perspectives of Medically Unexplained Symptoms. J. Psychosomatic Research. 54 (3), 215-218)

Chapter 4

Somatization: The Conversion of Mind into Matter, Psyche into Soma (Greek, body)

"The sorrow that has no vent in tears may make other organs weep." — Henry Maudsley

Julia is a 73-year-old woman with severe burning pain in her face. She has seen many physicians and has been diagnosed with "atypical facial pain". She has had multiple investigations and multiple treatments to no avail. On examination, she appears to be in no distress; in fact, she even appears jovial despite admitting to a level 10 pain. Several years ago, before her symptoms commenced, she had been a passenger in a car driven by her son. He crashed into a parked semi-truck in the darkness and was firmly wedged under the chassis. The car caught fire, Julia managed to escape, but her son could not and was burned to death. Her facial pain began shortly thereafter. She refuses to talk about the horrific incident but immediately refers to the facial pain. In some mysterious way, she has bodified her grief and brings it to the doctor. What a remarkable trick!

Somatization, bodifying, that process by which emotions are felt in the body, is normal. It is the way our brain functions, it is how we are "wired". Our brain is modular, different modules coming along at different periods in our evolution and they are not always fully integrated. Emotions reside in the older limbic brain, which is preverbal. Its theater of actions is the body, its language is the cramp in the guts, the misery of migraine, the iron grip of back and neck muscles. Only when [i]emotions are examined under the light of cognition, in the cortex, can we actually "feel". According to noted neuroscientist, Antonio Damasio, emotion plus language equals feeling. We can talk about our feelings, but our emotions take us to the doctor.

Our everyday language is suffused with bodily references to express emotion. The heart has top billing when it comes to translating emotion into bodily sensations:

- Heart of gold, broken-hearted, lighthearted, heavy-hearted, hard-hearted, soft-hearted, we "set our hearts" to a task, feel "from the bottom of our hearts", we even record "by heart" (Latin "cor" heart, re-cordire, by the heart), love you with all my heart. (Sadly, throughout human history, it has never been recorded that someone said, "I love you with all my brain".)

The gastrointestinal system is next in line:

- Gut feelings, knots in the stomach, butterflies in the belly, sinking feeling in the gut. You have guts if you are brave and gutless if you are not. If you are troublesome, you are an a…hole! Other organs are less frequently enlisted, but when you are angry, your blood is boiling, when you are a coward, you are spineless or lily-livered.

In one of the most provocative books of the 20th century, "The Origins of Consciousness in The Breakdown of The Bicameral Mind", Julian Jaynes, postulates that humans were not fully conscious until 3-4,000 years ago. He theorized that preconscious humans had no internal feelings; there was no "me" to narrativize thoughts and feelings. They used bodily sensations to convey emotion. This physical expression of emotions allowed individuals to communicate their internal states to others more effectively. As consciousness evolved, its ability to reflect on and articulate internal experiences became more pronounced. Now, for better or worse, modern humans can discuss and share their feelings, but most of the time, like our ancient ancestors, we emote rather than feel.

Allow me to give you an example of the bicameral mind in action. The following is taken from the sports section of the Los Angeles Times, Nov. 6, 1989. The writer is a wonderful example of what a preconscious sportswriter might have penned three thousand years ago.

Los Angeles Times, Nov. 6, 1989. Pro-Football: In a repeat of a disheartening loss at Buffalo, L.A. blows the lead and loses in overtime, 23-21.

Minneapolis – The Rams swore they would never forget Buffalo, and the memories of a last-minute loss on Oct. 16 that stuck to their insides like clumps of oatmeal, a taste so bitter it could not be duplicated, a feeling so strong it could not be tolerated.

The Rams wore the wounds of that loss, a gut-wrencher of ulcer-raising proportion, like lockets around their necks, hoping it would remain close to their hearts and serve as a warning to a game's funny bounces and its sometimes-humorless conclusions. (*The writer, Chris Dufresne, is obviously in touch with his emotions, if not his feelings.)*

Antonio Damasio: The Feeling of What Happens. Harcourt Brace. 1999

Charles V. Ford: Somatization and Fashionable Diagnoses: Illness as A Way of Life. Scan J. Work Envir. Health. 1997; 23 Supp 3: 7-16

De Gucht: Somatization: A Critical Psychosomatics Review. 43:1 Jan-Feb. 2002

J. Jaynes: The Origins of Consciousness in the Breakdown of the Bicameral Mind. Houghton Mifflin. 1976.

Chapter 5

When Somatization Becomes Sickness

It is easy to see that there is no huge chasm between the normal somatizing, which is how we express emotions, and somatization as a disorder. It achieves "disorder" status when it becomes an entrenched behavior and when illness becomes a way of being. Bodifying can be employed in a variety of ways. A patient might adopt an illness strategy, either as a means of communication or a coping strategy. (The atypical facial pain lady; it is easier for her to deal with facial pain than to face the horror of her son's death.) It could be a mechanism for eliciting support and care from others. Being a patient confers dignity and avoids the stigma of the "psychological". Michael Balint (1896-1970), a Hungarian psychoanalyst, wrote *"a medical diagnosis transforms unorganized illness, an agglomeration of complaints and symptoms that may be unclear, unconnected and mysterious, into an entity that is a more understandable, organized illness"*. Charles Lamb, famous 19th century essayist, wrote, "to be sick is to enjoy monarchal privileges." Symptoms and motives may vary, but the underlying phenomenon is the same: life problems, grief, greed and every other human dilemma expressed in the language of the body.

There is a darker side to somatization when it overlaps with malingering, where illness may at times be used to influence others, including loved ones. While important to acknowledge, this is not the focus here and is far less common than the presentations discussed throughout this book.

Somatization, somatization disorder, conversion disorder, functional neurological disorder, are different points on the spectrum of *bodifying*. This process is almost always below the level of awareness, for some a default mode of expressing discontent, for others a more profound need to transform distress into physical symptoms which are more bearable. As physicians, we often have to decode our patients' "body language" if we are to be effective healers.

Perhaps, thousands of years from now, we will be more "Mr. Spock-like" with fully integrated brains and a prefrontal cortex as the master conductor over the whole ensemble, but for now, we are hybrid creatures, a confusing blend of emotion, feeling and thinking.

"We are fragmented beings who cement ourselves together, but there are always cracks. Living with the cracks is part of being, well, reasonably healthy" ... — Siri Hustvedt

Balint M. The Doctor, His Patient, and The Illness. 1957

Chapter 6
Hypochondria and Alexithymia

Hypochondria and alexithymia are extreme examples of the *canalization* of emotions into physical symptoms. (Kreiden)

Hypochondria

Hypochondria is a rich source of medically unexplained symptoms. Between 3 and 6% of patients seen by primary care physicians suffer from hypochondria, the irrational fear of illness. These are the "worried well" and typically feel insulted by any suggestion that it's "all in their head". In the United States, it is estimated that $20 billion a year is spent on patients whose psychological distress leads to expensive and unnecessary tests and procedures. History is replete with stories of famous hypochondriacs. James Boswell, in his "Life of Johnson," recounts his subject's incessant complaints about his health, referring to hypochondria as "the English disease."

David is a 42-year-old successful executive who sees me once every four to six weeks for his latest disease. The last fatal illness was Huntington's disease, and before that, he survived multiple sclerosis. Predictably, he has amassed an impressive compilation of MRIs and CT scans. Now he is convinced he has ALS and indeed he has developed fasciculations, muscle twitches, that are a feature of that awful disease, in his case, however, they are of no significance. I have reassured him and performed the necessary simple tests, all of which are normal, but I know he will be back.

His no-nonsense family doctor told him that he is a hypochondriac. His psychologist has told him that he is "catastrophizing". His psychiatrist told him that he has generalized anxiety disorder and prescribed low-dose Prozac, but David is too anxious to take his anti-anxiety medication!

Hypochondria is also an ancient disorder mentioned in the writings of Hippocrates. The word means "below the ribcage". Greek, hypo, (below), chondros, (rib), and referred to digestive disorders of the organs "below the rib cage", the liver and stomach. In the 17th century, it was identified as linked to melancholy and was a fashionable diagnosis in its day. Oddly enough, it affected more men than women, perhaps a male version of hysteria, although today the few studies on the topic do not show a strong gender bias. It wasn't until the 19th century that hypochondria became synonymous with excessive fear of illness. It is yet another example of brain-body disorders. The hypochondriac is not imagining or hallucinating, they simply cannot filter out the normal noise of the body. The occasional skipped heartbeat, the normal pulsations of blood vessels in their ears when they lie down to sleep, the little lymph gland in the neck, and the occasional twitch of muscle are all magnified and elevated to threat level. They simply lack a normal filter (or they have a hypervigilant amygdala!)

One of the most dreaded diseases is amyotrophic lateral sclerosis, ALS. When studying this particular disease, many of my classmates, me included, developed fasciculations, that muscle twitching which can be a sign of ALS. It was not imaginary, but an example of how psychology _*is*_ *biology.*

Alexithymia

James is a 61-year-old engineer, He suffers from headaches, indigestion, and a host of other maladies. He regularly produces a current list of complaints that expands with every visit. In a recent visit, he recited the sad news of his wife's passing. I asked him how he is coping with his loss. He replied, "My headaches are out of control." Alexithymia is an extreme example of emotional compartmentalization. It is characterized by difficulty in identifying, understanding and expressing one's emotions. The name is derived from Greek words meaning "cannot read mood". The alexithymic simply cannot read their emotions.

Emotions are expressed as physical sensations, like the preconscious human of Julian Jaynes. Trying to elicit feelings from such a patient is like trying to squeeze blood from a stone. These patients are easy to deal with, very compliant and almost robotic in demeanor. It is more common in men. It is not so much a disorder, as it is a residue of our preconscious past when the emotional circuits did not "speak" to the cortex.

Conversion, somatoform, and hypochondriasis are variations on the theme of mind into body, that universal phenomenon whereby psychic distress is transformed into physical symptoms. It's the way we're wired!

Balint, M. "The Basic Fault". 1968

Chapter 7

Hysteria

"If the uterus lodges in the loins, the woman feels a hard lump or ball in her side, but when it mounts as high as the head, it causes pain around the eyes and nose, the head feels heavy, and drowsiness and lethargy set in."
— Hippocrates, c. 460-370 BC

The history of mysterious, ill-defined disorders is the history of hysteria. The vast majority of those afflicted are female. The very word *hysteria* is derived from the Greek *hysteros*, meaning uterus. This is a contentious topic involving sex (biology) and gender (culture). Medical doctors argue that the female body experiences more varieties of distress, but it is likely that an examination of the role of females in a male-dominated, patriarchal society offers a more plausible explanation. Illness can be a retreat from oppression and an effective weapon, albeit a passive and often self-destructive one. The sick, pallid, languishing female has long been a cherished symbol for 19th-century poets and artists. For the Victorian gentleman, an invalid wife was a status symbol. Victorian mothers' advice to their daughters on the matter of sex: "Close your eyes and think of England." One cannot understand these perplexing and ever-changing disorders without some appreciation of the role of women in society and their response to the patriarchy. The medical establishment has long been silent on the feminization of these puzzling, medically unexplained disorders. It has been left to feminist writers to explore this anomaly.

The ancient healers, all men, blamed the uterus for all female complaints. They believed the uterus refused to stay in its normal position and wandered around the body, creating mischief. The offending uterus was usually coaxed back into place with sweet-smelling perfumes near the vagina and foul-smelling, nauseating concoctions near the mouth. It was also believed that inducing sneezing would force the uterus back into position. Throughout the centuries, hysteria persisted, ever-changing in its manifestations, but always remaining the woman's provenance. The symptoms of hysteria included coughs, hiccups, tremors, tics, swooning, and convulsions, just about every symptom imaginable. The cure? Pregnancy!

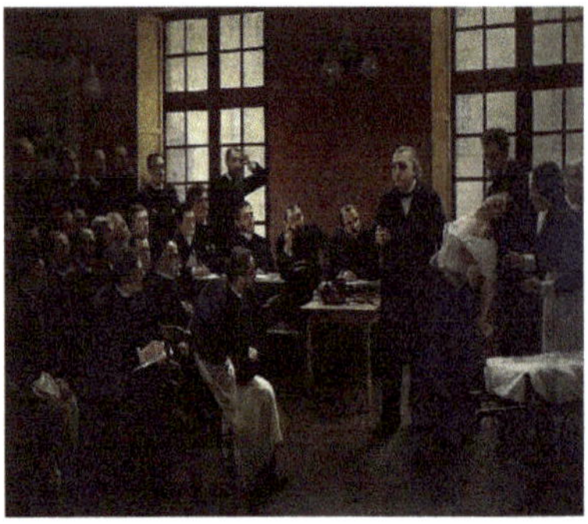

FIGURE 2: CHARCOT DEMONSTRATING HYSTERIA AT THE SALPETRIERE, 1887 (ANDRE BROUILLET)

Hysteria reached its high point (or low point) in France in the late 19th century. In the 1870s, Jean Marie Charcot, a brilliant neurologist and showman with great theatrical flair, instituted two weekly "performances" at the Salpêtrière Hospital to demonstrate "the grand hystérie." He hypnotized female patients and provoked hysterical fits for a fascinated male public, which included some of the most prominent physicians of the day. The female patients demonstrated bizarre postures and "fits," which the great maestro would showcase to a distinguished audience. It was very likely that these patients were coached in their exotic performances. Charcot became known as "the Napoleon of neurosis." Charcot, and later Freud, defined hysteria purely as a symptom of female sexual disorder when it was more likely a symptom of male sexual disorder! For the "patients," performing sexual hysterics for a titillated male audience was one opportunity for approval and a kind of fame. Charcot, a giant in the history of neurology, sullied his reputation with these theatrics. However, it was left to Sigmund Freud to initiate the schism between neurology and psychiatry.

Freud

Sigmund Freud, a student of Charcot, became disenchanted with his instructor's pyrotechnics. He was impressed by the "talking cure" devised by Joseph Breuer, a physician colleague who had successfully treated his patients using this method. Freud adopted the technique and soon it became identified with him, Dr. Breuer becoming a footnote in the annals of psychiatry. Freud shifted from neurology to an illness that could be treated with a psychological approach. For a neurologist accustomed to dealing with incurable, irreversible, degenerative diseases, the lure of a reversible disorder that responded to "talk treatment" was hard to resist. It paid off.

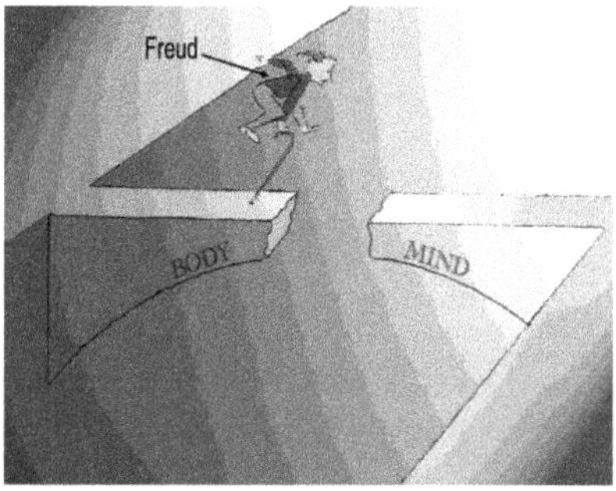

Freud understood that his psychoanalytic method lacked the serious stamp of science, but he realized that finding a physiological basis of psychological and mental disorders in the brain was a long way off. He had tried in 1895 with the *Project for Scientific Psychology*, but he abandoned it quickly, as did others who tried to find the basis for mental illness in specific brain regions. He wrote, *"The deficiencies in our psychoanalytic description would probably vanish if we were already in a position to replace the psychological terms with physical or chemical ones."* He knew that the mind and brain affected the body, but he lacked the *mechanistic link*; he called it "the puzzling leap." Abandoning the medical model, he and his followers left neuroanatomy and neuropathology behind, venturing into the sea of subjectivity and Mind.

The division between neurology and psychiatry became starkly clear: what was visible under the microscope was "neurology," and what was not was "psychiatry." It is fortunate that Freud abandoned his attempt at a brain science because it allowed him to develop descriptions of mental processes not based on experimental observation or contingent on vague correlations with neural mechanisms. He gave us the mind, not the brain, with profound insights that remain valid to this day. Perhaps his most enduring insight is the notion that inner conflicts, unrecognized by the person, can give rise to abnormal behaviors. Unfortunately, he also succumbed to "paradigm paralysis," with his brilliant insights fossilizing into a quasi-religious dogma that tolerated no deviation from the canon. His most brilliant pupil, Carl Gustav Jung, became an apostate by rejecting the central hypothesis of the Freudian creed, namely, sexual repression as the cause of every neurosis. The rift between medicine and psychiatry had begun, another manifestation of the mind-body split, known as dualism, the worm at the core of Western philosophy and science.

Edward Shorter: From Paralysis to Fatigue. The Free Press. 1993.
Elaine Showalter: Hystories. Columbia Press. 1997
Mark S. Micale: Approaching Hysteria. Princeton University Press. 1995

Chapter 8
Dualism and the Medical Model

"Alas dear God, there are two souls beating in one breast." — Goethe

"It is certain that this 'me,' that is to say my soul by which I am what I am, is entirely and absolutely distinct from my body and can exist without me."
— René Descartes, *Meditations VI*, 1641

Descartes is blamed for the concept of dualism, but in reality, we are all dualists. Daily, I hear patients comment as if their body is a separate entity, such as, "I was beside myself" (think how strange that sounds), or "My body is letting me down," "I want to but my body won't let me," or "My body is a mess," as if they are referring to an old automobile rusting in the garage. The playwright Tom Stoppard exclaimed, "I am not my body, my body is nothing without me."

In the language of philosophers, dualism is a concept that posits the existence of two distinct and fundamentally different types of realities. It is most commonly discussed in the context of the mind-body relationship, where it suggests that the mind and body are separate entities with different properties and functions. The mind is thought to be non-physical, associated with thoughts, consciousness, and emotions, while the body is physical and subject to physical laws. According to this concept, a person is composed of a body and soul, soma and psyche. The conscious psyche, or spirit, is imprisoned in the body as in a tomb but is independent of the body and survives after the body dies. (In Greek, *soma* means "body," but it can also mean "corpse" or "tomb.")

From Plato to the present, this mind-body dualism has been expressed in many ways. For Epictetus, mentor to Marcus Aurelius (of Gladiator fame), a human being is "a poor soul burdened with a corpse." Emperor Hadrian regarded his psyche like a beloved pet that he had to abandon when he died, "Dear little wandering lovely soul, you pale little thing, naked and stiff, into what regions will you now depart?" In more modern times, the Heaven's Gate cult, which committed mass suicide in San Diego years ago, wrote in their suicide notes that "they were exiting the vehicle", the "vehicle" being their useless, cumbersome body. The idea that mind and body are separate is as old as consciousness. The notion that there is a soul or spirit that outlives the mortal body is deeply intuitive and comforting, just as was the notion that the earth is flat and that the sun revolves around the earth.

Why this disconnect between psyche and soma? Mental life appears to stand in opposition to an objectified body that is being perceived from a distance, being repelled or solely experienced as a source of pain. There is no integral relationship between the mental and the somatic.

Perhaps it is due to the emergence of consciousness. The duality that has plagued us for millennia is not between mind and body but between consciousness and everything else. Being conscious allows us to see ourselves as discrete entities, as if from a distance, creating the illusion of separation between the "me" and "my body." We are aware of being aware; we can think about thinking. But consciousness may be an accident, an emergent property of billions of neurons and trillions of synapses trapped in a skull, and we are its slaves.

For doctors and patients, this mind-body dilemma is not some philosophical or theological conundrum. It affects our mental and physical health. It is present in every medical diagnosis, unspoken and unquestioned. Is it real or psychological? It influences the decisions made by insurance companies and governments regarding healthcare coverage. It has had devastating consequences for mental health disorders and has cost untold billions of dollars in the search for disease because it has made us blind to the contribution of the mind. This is one of the most costly and spurious dilemmas in the history of humanity.

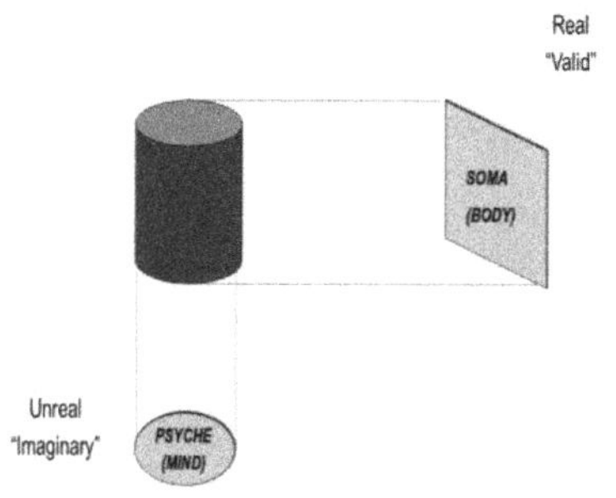

FIGURE 3: THE WILL TO MEANING (VICTOR FRANKL, 1969)

The mind-body dilemma, as it relates to the medical model, is perfectly captured in the cylinder model expressed by Viktor Frankl, a psychiatrist who survived the Nazi death camps. A person is depicted as a three-dimensional entity, like a cylinder. When illuminated horizontally, it appears as a rectangle, and when illuminated vertically, as a circle. Neither image captures the holism of the cylinder. In this metaphor, the person is divided into body (soma) and mind (psyche), and the two are separate.

To extend the metaphor, doctors take care of bodies, and psychiatrists take care of minds. There is an underlying innuendo, however: body problems are real, but "psych" problems are unreal, imaginary, and even a sign of moral weakness. Hence, the admonition to "go see a psychiatrist" is not only often unhelpful but also perceived as dismissive and insulting. At its worst, being referred for psychiatric care can be interpreted as a judgment of personal weakness or moral failing. This perception has deep historical roots. During the Spanish Inquisition, severe depression was often viewed as evidence of sinful behavior or character flaws. Individuals suffering from mental illness were sometimes believed to be under the influence of evil or divine punishment, and in extreme cases, they were subjected to brutal persecution.

The patient population is also a victim of the "real versus psychological" dilemma. They want validation, and they want a "real" diagnosis. They resist any psychological or behavioral contribution to their illness and insist on tests and procedures that may have already been performed multiple times.

Joan is a 33-year-old woman with a long history of chronic pain, fatigue, and brain fog. Her childhood was a nightmare of abuse and neglect. She has recently developed an eating disorder due to a feeling that there is some obstruction to the passage of food, but all tests are negative. She has become emaciated. She has a history of recurrent depression and anxiety, but has stopped all psychotropic medications in favor of natural healing. I spent a considerable amount of time explaining the link between depression, pain, and the eating disorder, and I thought I had made a breakthrough in the life of this unfortunate woman. She stormed out of my office, stating, "I have never been so insulted in my life." Beware the stigma of the "psych."

Insurance companies are also subject to the same delusion. They are more likely to spend the healthcare dollar on event-based, procedural medical interventions than pay for much-needed psychological support.

Eve is a 35-year-old woman with chronic daily headaches. She has undergone every conceivable test and treatment, including several spinal surgeries. Nothing has worked for her. Her childhood was an unimaginable horror; her crack-addicted mother traded her child's body for cocaine. Somehow, Eve survived but is now addicted to opioids in ever-increasing quantities. I requested a period of counseling for Eve, but it was rejected by the insurance company. The physician on my peer-to-peer phone interview said, "We don't cover psych." No doubt, Eve will continue to receive useless interventions from her pain physicians and yet another surgery because the medical model "doesn't cover psych."

Reflections on Mortality

An unfortunate consequence of being conscious is awareness of our mortality. We know that no matter how much we exercise, eat all the right foods, and take all the popular supplements, the goal of self-preservation will eventually be defeated. The stiffness in the joints, the nagging low-back pain, the crepe-like skin, sagging breasts, and flagging libido are constant reminders of our final destination. (That does not deter newly minted tech billionaires from trying. Longevity is now the goal, after the Gulf Stream jet and the private island. After all, what's the purpose of great wealth if one can't live forever?) The author William Styron expressed the forlorn hope, one that we all nurture in the depths of our being, "I've always known that everybody dies, but I've always thought that an exception would be made in my case." He was wrong.

Psychoanalyst Irvin Yalom describes our existential dilemma:

"The primitive dread of death resides in the unconscious, a dread that is part of the fabric of being, formed early in life before the development of precise conceptual formulation, a dread that is chilling, uncanny, and inchoate, a dread that exists prior to and outside of language and image."

Our answer to this awful dilemma is dualism. (We didn't have to invent it; it is the inevitable consequence of consciousness.) My body may die, but "I" live on. It is the body that betrays us, and so it should be punished. Throughout the long saga of human history, we have tortured and deprived the unfortunate body to liberate the psyche. Ascetics of all religions have devised novel ways to punish the body and reject bodily pleasures to achieve enlightenment, nirvana, satori, or Heaven!

Some of the early Christian ascetics, the Desert Fathers, abandoned civilization to live alone in the desert. Some took the novel step of castrating themselves lest they succumb to the pleasures of the flesh. However, this was frowned upon by the church authorities; it was considered a little too extreme. Equally extreme was Simeon the Stylite, who punished his rebellious body by living 36 years on a small platform atop a pillar. The most creative was the 5th-century monk who found the application of a small desert snake to his genitals a useful aid in his battle against masturbation.

This attitude towards the body has most definitely changed. Now, the body is venerated, celebrated, cosseted, and surgically altered in a never-ending quest for beauty, but it is still seen as separate from the "me." In our consumer culture, where individuals feel pressured to conform to specific beauty standards or lifestyles, the body is viewed as a product that can be packaged, sold, and sexualized, further detaching it from personal identity.

SOMA: Meaning in Homer. Calif Studies in Clinical Antiquity. Vol. 12. 1979. P. 269-282

Irv Yalom. 2008. Staring at the Sun: Overcoming the Terror of Death

Chapter 9
The Brain Gets in The Picture

"Men ought to know that from nothing else but the brain come joys, delights, laughter and sports, and sorrows, griefs, despondency and lamentations..." — Hippocrates

The medical model not only ignores the mind, but it also neglects the brain. It is an extraordinary fact that the organ which has propelled us to the top of the evolutionary ladder features so minimally in our understanding of human suffering. Nobody disputes that the brain is the central player in conventional diseases such as strokes, brain tumors, or Alzheimer's disease, but for many of the medically unexplained disorders, it scarcely features at all. To understand this extraordinary oversight, we need to look back in time. As Theodosius Dobzhansky observed, "nothing in Nature can be understood except from an evolutionary perspective."

In early organisms, there was no brain, only a few scattered collections of nerve cells called ganglia. Over the course of millions of years, these discrete bundles of cells began to coalesce into a single brain, its complexity growing to guide and control increasingly complex bodily systems. It became more complex, heavier, and more metabolically demanding. The brain became an energy hog, consuming 20% of our daily calories and oxygen, even though it accounts for only 2% of body weight. Eventually, it became so vital for the survival of the organism and so complicated in structure that it required special protection, retreating behind a fortress of bone like a feudal baron, surrounded by a moat, the blood-brain barrier. Access was jealously guarded, with passage guaranteed only to a select few.

To the ancients, and even to modern humans, the brain was a remote, mysterious organ, viewed with a mix of curiosity, reverence, and misunderstanding. In the Egypt of the Pharaohs, the brain was considered unimportant compared to other organs. During mummification, it was removed and discarded, while the heart was preserved, as it was believed to be the seat of intelligence and emotion.

For Hippocrates and the ancient Greeks, the brain was the seat of thought and sensation. (The great Aristotle, however, believed that the heart was the center of intellect, relegating the brain to a cooling organ for the blood). Despite our current understanding of the brain, it remains a subject of fascination and awe. In a piece of brain tissue the size of a grain of sand, there are over a hundred thousand neurons linked together by miles of wiring. One of the most notable differences between neurons and most other cells in the body is the intricate, weblike processes called dendrites, which receive signals from millions of other neurons.

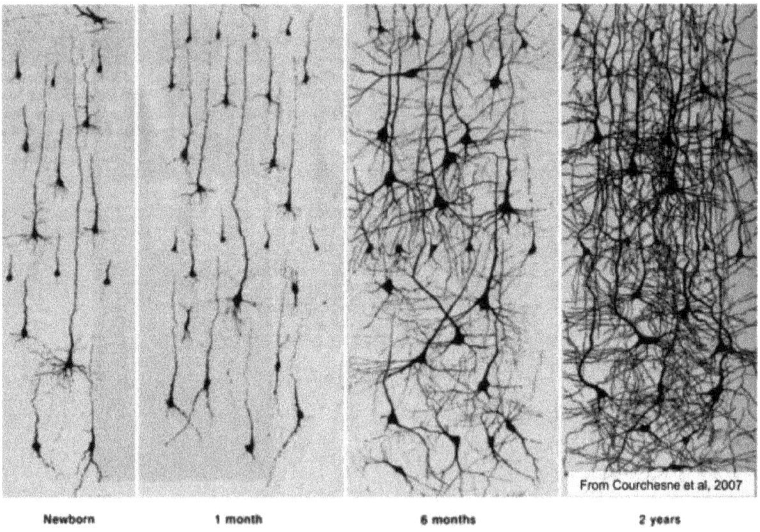

The neurons in Einstein's brain are the same as those in a mouse brain, but Einstein had many more of them, between 80 and 100 billion, as do all humans, with trillions of synaptic connections to other neurons. From these humble biological bits emerges… MIND. *Emergence is the way complex systems arise out of a*

multiplicity of simple interactions: the ant colony is a masterpiece of organization, but we will never understand the ant colony by examining an individual ant. The neuron or brain cell is analogous to the ant, by itself capable of only the simplest function, but pack 80 billion of them into a skull with a few trillion connections, and mind emerges. It's a miracle! (But miracles are just nature unexplained... Spinoza.)

This is the materialist view of mind to which I subscribe. There are serious thinkers who feel that the mind/consciousness is independent of the brain. They hypothesize that our brains are like our iPhones that lock into a universal consciousness. These philosophers should spend a few days in a brain rehab center! Patricia Churchland, a "sensible" philosopher, states that saying the brain has nothing to do with consciousness is like saying the heart has nothing to do with circulation.

Dualism Vs. Trialism

Mind, a mysterious matter secreted by the brain. Its chief activity consists in the endeavor to ascertain its own nature, the futility of the attempt being due to the fact that it has nothing but itself to know itself with. Ambrose Bierce

The problem of Dualism is really "Trialism." We can reduce the mind-body problem to the mind-brain problem and the brain-body problem. As to the former, we should leave it to philosophers to ponder how 3 pounds of electrified jelly give rise to Mind, Mozart, and Charles Manson. In philosophy, this is referred to as the "hard problem", i.e., how does subjective conscious experience emanate from physical brain states? Our concern as physicians is the brain-body connection. We must sidestep the mind for the moment and emphasize brain-body communication. Of course, much human misery results from an inability to cope, poor choices, and bad habits, rather than any failure of brain components, but "normal" misery is not our concern. The focus of this book is those conditions that have assumed "MUD status," where presumably there is alteration in brain structure and function, leading to a more entrenched state. This is a more refined form of reductionism, but one that is supported by neuroscience and more acceptable to the patient.

The Brain-Body Connection

We now have the neuroscience to explain how severe mental stress, especially in childhood, causes distinct changes in brain circuits that are fundamental to the development of many medically unexplained disorders. We have enough neurobiology to bridge the "puzzling leap," at least in some of these disorders. It is pitifully incomplete, but better than vague, convoluted psychoanalytic theories. People can understand and accept brain disorders more than "mind disorders" with their innuendo of weakness and degeneracy, reminiscent of 19th century thinking. In many medically unexplained disorders, the brain changes may be primary, although it is often impossible to separate mind from brain. I propose a neologism, THE BRAIND! At least this term captures the futility of trying to separate brain and mind.

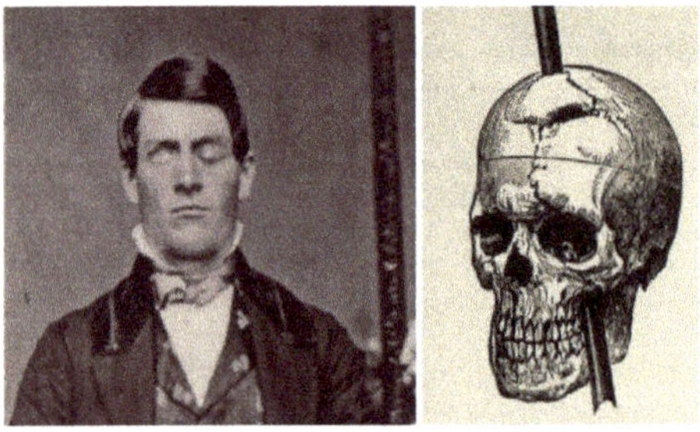

FIGURE 4: HARVARD MEDICAL MUSEUM

There have been many occasions throughout history where the apparent separation between mind and body has been shattered, none more famous than the case of Phineas Gage. In 1848, he was a 25-year-old railroad engineer in Vermont. One day, while using a tamping iron to pack explosive powder into a hole, an accidental explosion occurred. The tamping iron, a three-foot-long heavy metal rod, was propelled through the air, striking Gage in the head. The rod entered his left cheek and exited through the top of his head, damaging the frontal lobes of the brain. Miraculously, he survived the accident and was able to walk and talk shortly afterward. However, the most significant changes occurred in his personality. Before the accident, he was known to be responsible, sober, sociable, and well-liked. After the accident, he exhibited drastic changes in behavior. He became impulsive, irresponsible, profane, and prone to fits of rage. His friends and family stated he was no longer the same person.

We need no longer refer to the story of Phineas Gage to illustrate the fallacy of the mind-body separation. In more recent times, Dr. Walter Freeman (1895–1972), a psychiatrist, performed over 2,000 lobotomies using an ice pick, which he performed without gloves or masks. Many died, and others were left in a lobotomized state. One survivor said that he "had lost his soul." One of his most famous cases was the case of the sister of President John F. Kennedy. The procedure left her disabled, requiring lifelong institutionalization. Gustav Flaubert wrote, "You cannot find the soul with a scalpel, but you can destroy it with one."

It is the illusion of remoteness that has led us to think that the brain and body have little or no communication. Brain and body are engaged in constant bidirectional communication. The brain speaks to the body via an intricate web of nerves and chemicals, and the body maintains a constant flow of information to the brain via the vagus nerve and chemical messengers from the organs, especially the gut. Before we examine the intricate brain-body connectivity, it is very important to address some basic features of brain anatomy, especially those structures involved in the stress response.

Chapter 10

Brain 101

"The brain is an integrated evolved structure with different bits of it appearing at different moments in evolution and adapted to some different problems." — Francis Crick

In other words, the brain is not a single prepackaged entity; it is modular, composed of different parts that emerged at different periods of evolution, each new structure blending with the old. (One eminent neuroscientist says, "If you want proof of lack of intelligent design of the universe, look no further than the human brain.")

Paul MacLean (1913– 2007), a Harvard neurobiologist, formulated the so-called "triune brain" hypothesis. This tripartite theory is far from universally accepted by all neurobiologists, but it can serve as a useful model. Theories do not have to be right; they must be useful, and this model is very useful in helping us understand the basic organization of the human brain. The triune brain theory proposes that there are three major components of the modern human nervous system:

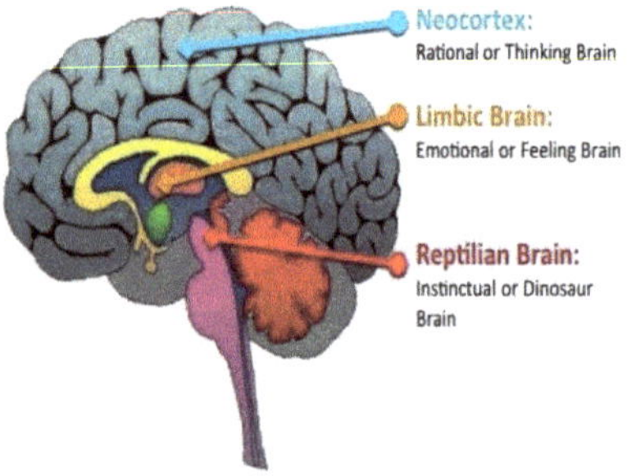

FIGURE 5: MACLEAN P.D. (1970). THE TRIUNE BRAIN IN EVOLUTION

The R Complex: Known as the reptilian brain, this includes the brainstem and cerebellum. Its purpose is bodily maintenance, such as breathing, blood flow, digestion, and other bodily functions. It is also responsible for primitive behaviors like aggression, dominance, and territoriality. In ancient brains, there were two structures that could be identified: the thalamus and the basal ganglia. The thalamus was mostly in charge of receiving and processing information from the external world, while the basal ganglia were responsible for movement and action. A few hundred million years later, the emotional brain — the limbic system — entered the picture.

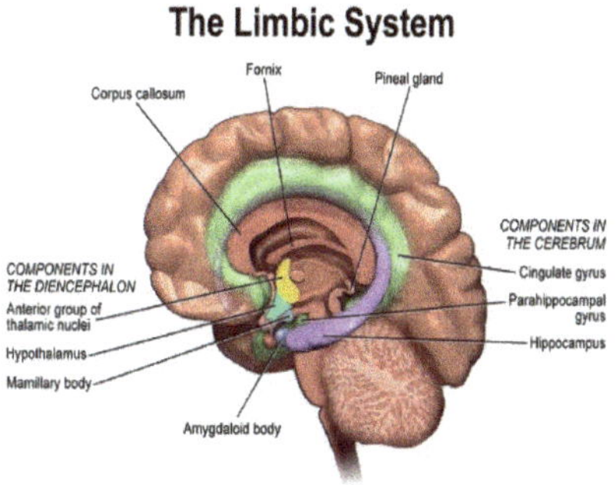

The Limbic System (The Emotional Brain): Derived from the Latin word *limbus*, meaning "border" or "edge," as it appeared to the ancient anatomists because it wrapped around the old brain structures. It includes the hippocampus, amygdala, cingulate cortex, and hypothalamus. It houses the primary centers of emotion. While we can point to these structures as "emotional centers," we still have no idea how neurons create emotions from experience, any more than we know how neurons create "mind." Shakespeare queried: "Tell me where is fancy bred, Or in the heart or in the head?" (*The Merchant of Venice*) We have made progress in 400 years. It's not in the heart!

The Hypothalamus: Closely linked to the thalamus, the hypothalamus monitors internal states and helps maintain balance within the organism, known as homeostasis. This tiny area, no larger than the nail on the little finger, regulates many vital functions such as eating, sleep-waking cycles, control of body temperature, and appetite. It is also the portal by which the emotional brain speaks to the rest of the body. There are two outflow pathways from the hypothalamus connecting the brain to every organ in the body, including the immune system. One pathway is the autonomic nervous system (ANS), and the other involves the synthesis and release of hormones into the pituitary and adrenal glands, known as the hypothalamic-pituitary-adrenal axis (HPAA). Both pathways are key players in the stress response.

The Autonomic Nervous System (ANS):

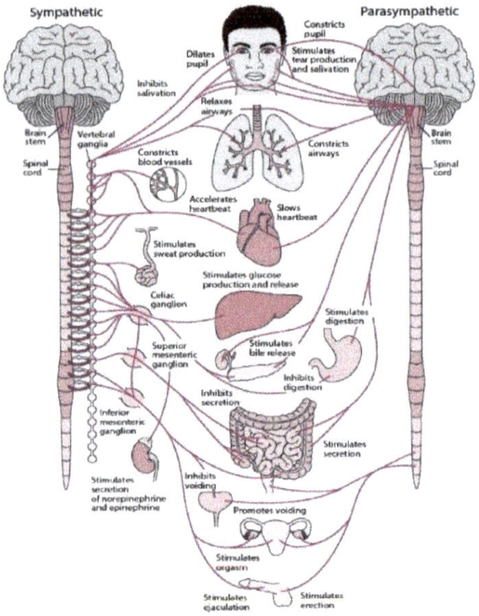

It is called autonomic, or automatic, because this specialized network of nerves controls bodily responses that are not under voluntary control. There are two general divisions within the ANS: the Sympathetic Nervous System (SNS), which, when activated, readies the body for action, and the Parasympathetic Nervous System (PNS), which acts as a countermeasure for the sympathetic division. Activation of the sympathetic division sharpens the senses, alerts the body to danger, and prepares it for fight-or-flight. The parasympathetic division acts as a counterbalance, slowing the heart rate, aiding digestion, and promoting relaxation and sleep. It is the "rest and digest" part of the system, allowing digestion and refilling of energy reservoirs.

The Vagus Nerve:

A major component of the parasympathetic nervous system, (vagus from the Latin *wandering*) plays a crucial role in regulating involuntary functions of the body, including heart rate, digestion, and respiratory rate. It was called “the Great Nerve” by Galen. It is the primary conduit for transmitting and

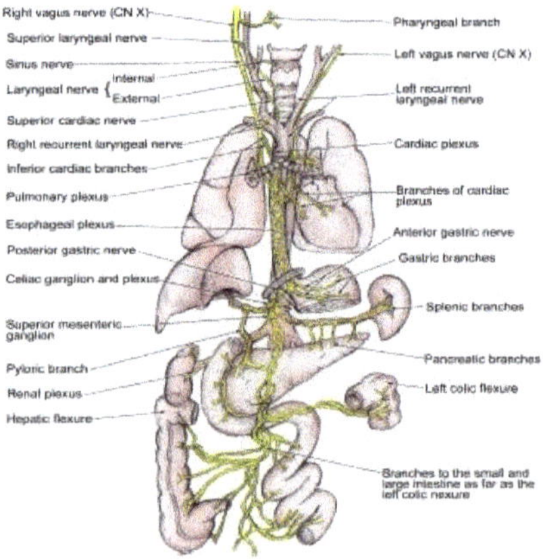

receiving signals between the brain and the organs, predominantly the heart and intestines.

The Hypothalamic-Pituitary-Adrenal Axis (HPAA):

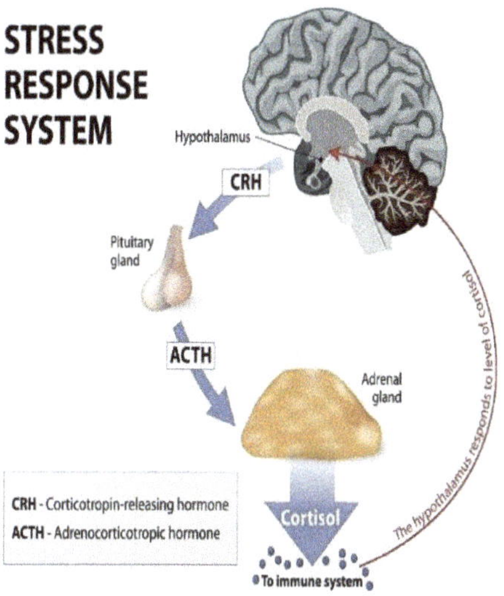

The HPAA is a complex network of interactions among three key components of the stress system: the hypothalamus, the pituitary gland, and the adrenal glands. This circuit plays a critical role in the body's response to stress. Several vital stress hormones are released via this system, including corticotropin-releasing factor (CRF), cortisol, and adrenaline.

The Amygdala:

The amygdala, an almond-shaped structure (Greek, *amygdalon* = almond), sits at the tip of both temporal lobes; it is our early warning radar system. It is critical in attaching emotional significance to all incoming sensory stimuli, not just the scary stuff. A lion roaring in a zoo provokes no fear, but if one is abandoned in the savannah alone, the sound strikes terror. It is our early warning radar system. Information about the outside world is transmitted to the amygdala, allowing it to monitor for signs of danger. When sensory information about a threatening stimulus is detected, output connections to response-control systems in the brainstem initiate the expression of defense responses and support physiological changes in the body.

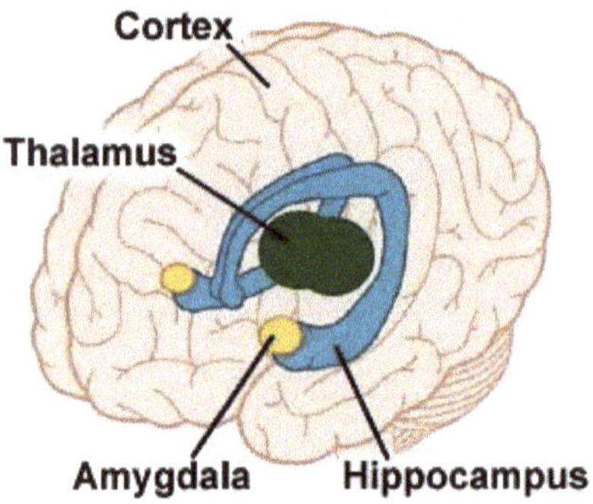

The amygdala does not act on its own; it is normally under the control of the prefrontal cortex and the hippocampus. This pathway acts to control and modify the amygdala's responses. Studies have shown that humans have more brain circuits going from the cortex back to the amygdala than any other species. Even so, under extreme stress, the amygdala may bypass this process and activate the full-blown fight-or-flight response, known as "amygdala hijack." The amygdala is the major actor in the stress response.

<u>The Hippocampus:</u>

The hippocampus is a small, curved structure within the brain's temporal lobe and is part of the limbic system. It plays a crucial role in various cognitive functions, particularly in the formation and retrieval of memories. As part of the limbic system, the hippocampus interacts with other brain regions involved in emotions. Via its connection with the prefrontal cortex, it exerts a powerful influence on the amygdala. The hippocampus is also critical in converting information into long-term memory and recall. (*Dr. Eleanor Maguire studied London taxi drivers, impressed by their prodigious memory capacity (before the advent of GPS). Her studies revealed that the hippocampus can actually grow. Neurogenesis, the formation of new brain cells, is essential for the formation of new memories. The posterior hippocampi of taxi drivers were significantly larger relative to those of control subjects. The longer the cabby had been a driver, the bigger the hippocampus. This key structure in the brain governing memory and spatial navigation was actually malleable. I shudder to think what is happening to the hippocampus of modern humans who have outsourced their navigation to their iPhone.*)

Because the hippocampus is so malleable, it is vulnerable to prolonged stress. Shrinkage of the hippocampus was one of the first visible brain changes in depression and PTSD and explains why depression is associated with "pseudo- dementia."

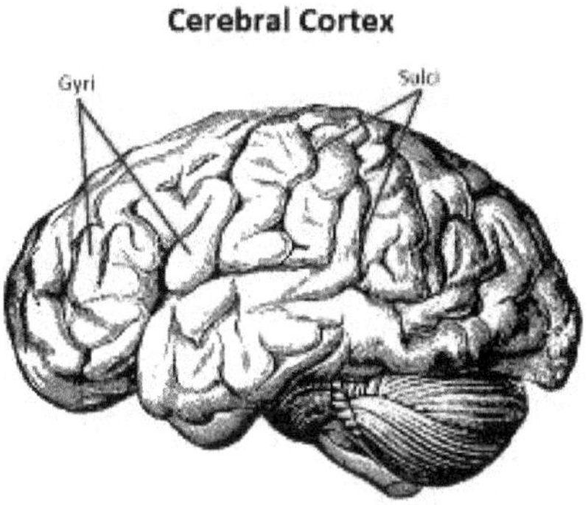

The Cortex: (Latin, *cortex* = bark, as in the bark of a tree). The name is appropriate since it wraps around all of the older brain structures. It is the last portion of the brain to appear and is what makes us uniquely human. The intrinsic qualities of the human cortex give us greater power of imagination than is available to other species. Logical reasoning, judgment, and planning for the future are functions of the cortex. One part of the cortex, the prefrontal cortex (PFC), is often referred to as the executive center or command post, as its main function is to control the older emotional brain, the limbic brain. Human beings depend on the formidable prefrontal cortex to overcome instinctive, amygdala-driven urges. The importance of this region can be seen when there is damage to this area, as in the case of Phineas Gage. He is a powerful example of what happens when the frontal cortex is damaged: emotions become out of control, and behavior is inappropriate and uninhibited. In fact, we don't need such an extreme example as Phineas Gage to tell us how fragile and tenuous the control of the cortex over the older brain structures is. A few glasses of alcohol, and a normally temperate individual may act in a disinhibited fashion, often to their great embarrassment once the effects of alcohol have passed.

Philosophers and sociologists have mused on the consequences of pairing these ancient, primitive brain structures with intelligence and planning. It makes us a very lethal species. We are the only species capable of industrialized killing. Perhaps Nietzsche had this in mind when he said, "There is a touch of evil in every living creature, but when God created man, he had the devil at his elbow."

The components of the stress response are in place. Now we will examine how these pieces fit together in response to threat and stress. It is this response that vividly illuminates the brain in action.

Maclean P.D. (1970). The Triune Brain in Evolution. NY Plenum Press.

Chapter 11

Stress

"Our defense mechanisms are designed for the 30-second struggle with the saber-tooth tiger, not for the 30-year marriage or the 30-year mortgage."
— Robert Sapolsky

"Our age of anxiety is the result of doing today's job with yesterday's tools and yesterday's concepts."
— Marshall McLuhan

Modern humans live in a technologically advanced and complex world, but we are still equipped with Stone Age brains when it comes to dealing with stress and the challenges of everyday life. Embedded in our nervous systems are neural programs that were adapted for a primitive hunter-gatherer, but in a sophisticated modern society, our stresses are chronic and ambiguous. Modern humans rarely have to engage the fight-or-flight response because of a threat from a predator. Hunger, war, or genocidal conflict are not the main threats for most of us. For us, the predator, sneaky and in multiple disguises, is stress, the stress of being human, of just living. Robert Sapolsky, neuroscientist and primatologist, has said that our stress is not the thirty-second struggle with the saber-toothed tiger, it is the 30-year marriage or the 30-year mortgage! However, even though our stress is psychosocial and chronic, we still activate the same circuitry as if we are fleeing from a predator.

Chronic stress plays a huge role in many different disease states, but is a dominant factor in medically unexplained disorders. (The biggest source of stress for most humans is fear of the negative reactions of other people. We evolved as a group species. On the savannah or in the jungle, to be an outcast from the group was death. In laboratory settings, where human stress responses are evaluated, speaking in front of a group is the maximum stressor.)

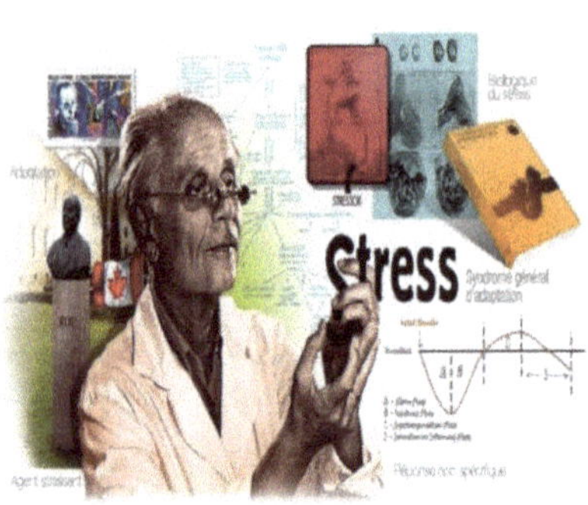

It is sobering to realize that the word "stress" did not exist in medical language until a brief paper by Hungarian physician Hans Selye, published in 1937, entitled "A Syndrome Produced by Diverse Noxious Agents." He did not invent the word "stress"; he borrowed it from engineers and metallurgists. Prior to that time, the concept of stress did not exist in medicine. Now, virtually every language in the world has its own word for stress (in French, Le Stress).

Selye was born in Vienna to Hungarian parents. Homeschooled, he was speaking four languages by age four, with more to come. During his medical training in Montreal, Canada, he noticed how professors adhered strictly to the medical model, often missing the "syndrome of just being sick." Selye was the first scientist to identify 'stress' as underpinning the nonspecific signs and symptoms of illness. He was seemingly immune to stress, publishing 1,600 journal articles and 40 books!

The Acute Stress Response

For the ancient hunter-gatherer confronting the saber-toothed tiger, there is no ambiguity. The threat is clearly identified, and the stress response system is activated. Visual information from the optic nerves is processed immediately, and signals are flashed to the amygdala. Its role is to evaluate the threat level and react accordingly. In the face of a definite threat signal, the amygdala activates the hypothalamus, which in turn activates the sympathetic nervous system (SNS) and the fight-or-flight response. The two outflow systems, the autonomic nervous system (ANS) and the hypothalamic-pituitary-adrenal axis (HPAA), are activated.

Phase One:
The Sympathetic Nervous System (SNS)

The SNS is responsible for the immediate stress response. There is an immediate outpouring of adrenaline with predictable results: heart rate increases, breathing becomes rapid to provide oxygen for the extra blood pumping through the body, skin grows pale as blood is diverted into the deep muscles, the mouth becomes dry, and the bowel and bladder may empty. (This makes tactical sense, getting rid of excess baggage and lessening the chance of infection if wounded or gored.) Adrenaline also provides an abundant supply of glucose, which is the high-octane fuel for the body. Glucose is stored in the liver in the form of glycogen. It is not immediately available for use until adrenaline stimulates the breakdown of glycogen, chopping molecules into glucose. Adrenaline also inhibits insulin release, allowing more glucose to enter the bloodstream. A recent study in Nature demonstrates that in acute stress, the amygdala directly communicates with the liver to elevate blood glucose.

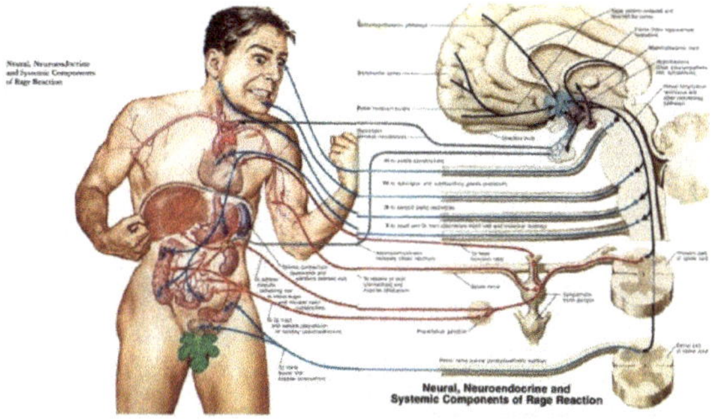

FIGURE 6: FRANK H. NETTER, MD, CIBA COLLECTION OF MEDICAL ILLUSTRATIONS, 1983

The SNS also communicates with the immune system, which is vital for the Department of Defense. White blood cells are marshaled from depositories in the bone marrow and spleen and sent into battle. The inflammatory response is initiated. Cytokines, messenger molecules released at the site of inflammation, recruit other immune cells and travel to the brain, ensuring the "Dept. of Defense" is informed of the situation downstream.

Phase Two: The Hypothalamic-Pituitary-Adrenal Axis (HPAA)

A little while later, lagging behind the adrenaline burst, the HPAA is activated. The same burst of signals from the amygdala activates cells in the hypothalamus, causing the release of a hormone called corticotropin-releasing factor (CRF). This molecule travels via a conduit of tiny vessels to the pituitary gland, which responds by secreting another hormone, adrenal corticotropic hormone (ACTH). This is released into the general circulation and travels to the adrenal glands, specifically the adrenal cortex, where cortisol is synthesized and released. The primary function of cortisol is to increase blood glucose levels through the breakdown of glycogen, which is a storage form of glucose. Cortisol's action is not as direct as adrenaline's, but it facilitates the process by ensuring a steady glucose supply.

Cortisol has immense importance in the body with several pivotal roles. In addition to facilitating the supply of glucose, it is also anti-inflammatory and immunosuppressive. It acts as a counterbalance to the pro-inflammatory and immune-activating effect of the sympathetic nervous system. Inflammation is a powerful two-edged sword, vital for the acute phase of the stress response, but devastating if left on too long. However, cortisol too can have ruinous effects if left unchecked, which is why it inhibits its own release via a negative feedback loop to the hypothalamus. (This is a wonderful example of the negative feedback loops that control biological systems: the regulator must also be regulated!)

Memory of the Encounter

Mercifully, our ancient ancestor survived the encounter with the saber-toothed tiger. The stress-response system, our Department of Defense, has done its job. The effect of the SNS has given him the extra blood, oxygen, and glucose fuel for his life-saving flight. The inflammatory response has been turned on, and the damaged areas are flooded with white blood cells and life-saving chemicals to fight infection. Cortisol is now also operating at full tilt, doing its mopping-up operation, limiting the inflammatory process, and helping to restore normalcy to the exhausted hunter. However, it is crucial for him to remember the circumstances of the encounter if he is to survive.

Memories are longer-lasting when the situation is arousing. In the presence of adrenaline, the consolidation of memory is enhanced. However, the more horrific the encounter — and the more adrenaline released — the more long-lasting the memory, and the more likely the development of post-traumatic stress disorder (PTSD). (In the modern era, soldiers going into battle are equipped with beta-blockers, which block the effect of adrenaline and hopefully prevent the formation of PTSD.)

This beautifully balanced, synchronized stress system operates optimally in response to short-term stressors. Our ancestor had no mortgage on his Stone-Age cave, nor was he being hounded for outstanding debt. His concern was for the immediate present. Hence, the stress response has evolved over brief periods of time, from seconds to hours. As we will see in the next chapter, when the stress is chronic and long-lasting, the effects can be detrimental, with potentially devastating consequences.

Hans Selye: "A Syndrome Produced by Diverse Noxious Agents". Nature. 1937

M. Joels: The Neurosymphony of Stress. Nat. Rev. Neuroscience. 2009. Vol. 10. 459-466

B. McEwan: The End of Stress as we Know It. Joseph Henry Press. 2004

R. Sapolsky: Behave. Penguin Press. 2017

M. Meaney: Ann. Review Neuroscience. 2001, 24; 1:161-192

M. Teicher: The Neurobiology of Childhood Stress. 2016

Chapter 12

When The Stress is Chronic

"Any idiot can deal with a crisis; it's the day-to-day stuff that wears you down". — Anton Chekhov

A certain amount of stress is inevitable. However, this delicately balanced, intricate stress response system was not designed for protracted long-term stress. When stress becomes chronic, there are devastating consequences for body and brain. With protracted stress, it is necessary to maintain the increased activity of the sympathetic nervous system (SNS) and the hypothalamic-pituitary-adrenal axis (HPAA, resulting in excess adrenaline and cortisol.

Overactivity of the SNS: Adrenaline Overdose

We are all aware of the intense physiological reactions when one is confronted by a sudden, terrifying event: the feeling of intense fear, sweating, rapid heart rate, increased breathing, tightening of muscles, etc., are all consequences of the initial adrenaline rush. When the stress becomes chronic, this system may be permanently fixed in the "on position" resulting in hypertension, coronary artery spasm and chronic anxiety (the main ingredient in most of the medically unexplained disorders)

Takotsubo, often referred to as the "broken heart syndrome" is a temporary heart condition that mimics the symptoms of a heart attack. First described in 1990 in Japan, takotsubo is a weakening of the left ventricle, the heart's main pumping chamber. The condition is usually the result of severe emotional or physical stress, that's why the condition is also called stress-induced cardiomyopathy or broken

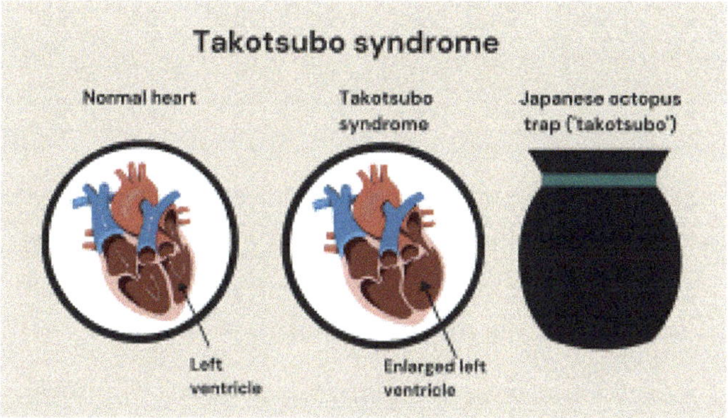

heart syndrome. The name takotsubo comes from the Japanese word for an octopus trap, as the shape of the heart during this condition resembles the vase-shaped trap that Japanese fishermen use to catch octopuses. Although the exact mechanism is not fully understood, it is believed that a surge of adrenaline can temporarily damage the heart muscle. It is interesting to note that 90% of reported cases are in women aged 58 to 75!

Overactivity of the HPAA:

There are two powerful hormones secreted by the HPAA: corticotropin-releasing factor (CRF) and cortisol.

CRF: Overactivity of CRF is one of the long-term neurobiological consequences of early life trauma and is a major risk for the development of mood disorders in later life. 25. With hypersecretion of CRF, there is a shift from normal attentiveness to a state of excitement and anxiety. Excess central CRF secretion has been implicated in many stress-related disorders, including depression and irritable bowel syndrome (IBS). Increased levels of CRF lead to increased cortisol output.

Cortisol is a central molecule in stress-related disorders. Since the early work of Hans Selye, it has been known that chronic stress may result in hypercortisolemia, an excess of cortisol. It is so potent that it must be kept within an optimal narrow range by an elaborate negative feedback system. There is a normal diurnal or daily variation of cortisol, but the range is tightly controlled in an individual subject. That the body would have such a tightly regulated control system suggests that excessive, unchecked activity could be detrimental to the organism. Excessive and sustained cortisol secretion has long been associated with depression, hypertension, immunosuppression, diabetes, osteoporosis and coronary artery disease. In all these disorders, stress triggers disease by increasing the output of cortisol, exposing the body to elevated concentrations of this hormone.

The paradox of the stress response lies in the simultaneity of its adaptive nature and its possible maladaptive consequences. (Marius Tausk, German physiologist, illustrated this paradox with his illustration of the fireman's hose. The water used to extinguish the fire may cause more damage than the fire itself. Like the fireman's water, stress responses are initially beneficial but can impose a cost to the body and brain when they are elicited too often). That burden is referred to as the allostatic load. This term, coined by Bruce McEwen, refers to the cumulative physiological wear and tear on the body that results from prolonged exposure to stress and the body's attempt to adapt to that stress. It's the "butcher's bill", the price we pay for being human in a world to which we have never fully adapted.[26]

The Stressed-out Brain:

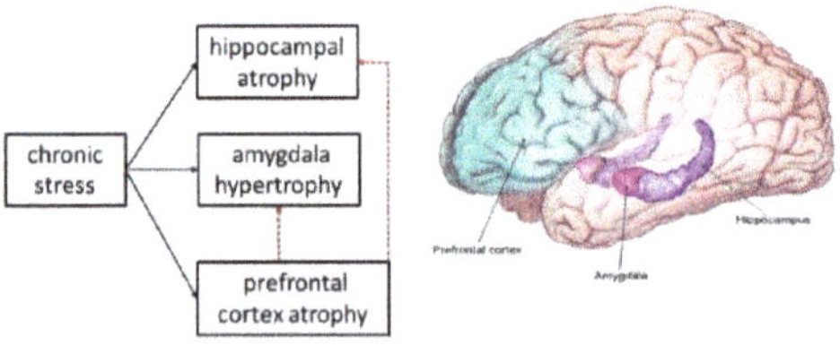

Long-term stress not only exacts a toll on the body but also on the brain. The hippocampus was the first brain area recognized as a major target of stress hormones. This hippocampus is one of the most sensitive and susceptible regions of the brain to chronic stress, precisely because it is malleable and ever-changing. High levels of cortisol, which occur in chronic stress, damage the hippocampus. As mentioned previously, the hippocampus and its connections with the prefrontal cortex exert potent negative feedback on the stress response. A damaged hippocampus leads to a less inhibited amygdala and a more powerful stress response, which then damages the hippocampus further, a vicious cycle: stress leads to hippocampal damage, which in turn leads to a heightened stress response.

Shrinkage of the hippocampus and its cortical connections have been the most reproducible findings in chronic stress regardless of whether the stress is from depression, PTSD or childhood abuse. Victims of sexual abuse show a 20% reduction in hippocampal volume. Other structures in the limbic system, such as the amygdala, also undergo structural remodeling, in the opposite direction, leading to a heightened response to all incoming sensory traffic.

"Experience, life and long-lasting stress all affect brain structure and function. The body keeps the score." — Bessel van der Kolk. Psychology IS Biology

McEwen B.S. (1998). Stress, Adaptation and Diseases: Allostasis and Allostatic Load. Annals of the NY Acad. of Sciences, 840 (1) 35-44.
Sapolsky, R.M. (2004). Why Stress is Bad for Your Brain. Science, 293 (5532), 512-513.
Chrousos, G.P. (2009). Stress and Disorders of the Stress System. Nature Reviews Endocrinology, 5 (7), 374-381.
When The Body Says No. Exploring The Stress Disease Connection. Gabor Mate. Trade Paper Press. 2003.

Chapter 13

Early Childhood / Adolescent Stress

"When I look back on my childhood, I wonder how I survived at all. It was, of course, a miserable childhood: the happy childhood is hardly worth your while. Worse than the ordinary miserable childhood is the miserable Irish childhood, and worse yet is the miserable Irish Catholic childhood."— Frank McCourt, Angela's Ashes

They f..k you up, your mum and dad
They may not mean to, but they do.
They fill you with the faults they had
And add some extra just for you

— Philip Larkin, This Be the Verse

Countless times while evaluating patients with chronic disorders, I have been impressed with the frequent history of childhood abuse and stress. There is little doubt that many of the medically unexplained disorders, especially chronic pain, have their genesis in early childhood and adolescent trauma.

Childhood in humans, or the early life period, is a pivotal period in development where much of the pain neurocircuitry is primed for lifelong function. More than 10% of children in the US report experiencing neglect or physical or psychological abuse. The long-term consequences on pain perception lead to chronic, unmanageable health problems. Studies by Martin Teicher, an adolescent and child psychiatrist at Harvard, have revealed the structural changes in the brain caused by adverse early life events. There is a thinner, smaller cortex with less gray matter in the brains of adults with early life stress. As noted, continuous exposure to high levels of stress hormones also alters the structure of vulnerable emotional circuits such as the amygdala and hippocampus. The hippocampus is weakened, leaving less restraint on the amygdala, which, in contrast, expands in size and becomes hyperactive. The emotional circuitry is no longer held in check by the higher centers. In such people, there is a tendency to face life challenges with anger, frustration and less inhibition of destructive emotions. These are the patients who haunt the headache centers, spinal clinics and pain centers.

Researchers have formulated a scoring system to try to quantify the severity of the abuse. With each increase in adverse childhood experience, there is an increase in the likelihood of a hyperactive amygdala and a sluggish prefrontal cortex that never fully developed, leading to distortion and amplification of all incoming sensations, including pain.

Noted neuroscientist, Antonio Damasio, expressed the same reality in his Somatic Marker Hypothesis. He theorizes that the hyperactivity of the amygdala, combined with the hypoactivity of the top-down control due to damage to a specific part of the prefrontal cortex, can trigger impulsivity, addiction and impaired decision-making.

Dr. Teicher expresses this tragic reality eloquently:

"Early abuse molds the limbic system to be more irritable, impulsive, suspicious, and prone to be swamped by fight or flight reactions that the cortex may not be able to control. To a brain so tuned, Eden itself would seem to hold its share of danger."

Meaney's Rats

The work of Teicher and others is truly groundbreaking and has dealt a deathblow to the mind-body dilemma. However, there is a need for a more fundamental understanding of how neural circuits in our brains are altered by chronic stress. For this knowledge, we must rely on animal studies, especially animal models of early life adversity.

The pivotal experiments began in 1980 under the direction of Michael Meaney at McGill University in Montreal. He is one of the most highly cited neuroscientists in the world. His team took genetically identical rat mothers, yet showing distinct differences in mothering style, some rat mommies were naturally nurturing and others were naturally negligent. The offspring of negligent mothers, stressed-out youngsters, grew into loners prone to the rat equivalent of anxiety and depression and addictive behaviors. When offered cocaine and alcohol, they binged.

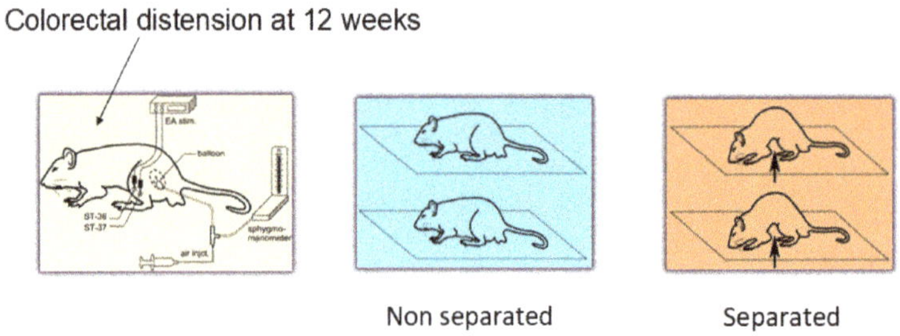

Another variant of the maternal separation model included the colonic distension model. This is widely used to study visceral pain responses in rats in the context of early life stress, such as maternal separation. This is particularly relevant for the understanding of chronic pain. In this model, newborn rats have a catheter inserted into the rectum at birth. Again, two distinct groups were formed, one group separated from the mommy at birth and the other group normally reared and pampered. When the catheter was inflated at the appointed time, the colon was distended, which is very painful. The maternally separated rat pups showed a markedly heightened sensitivity to pain compared with non-separated controls. They also exhibited anxiety-like behaviors and exaggerated responses to all stressors, including pain. Obviously, these findings have profound implications for the most common of all gastrointestinal disorders, irritable bowel syndrome IBS.

What was more remarkable were the insights into the biological mechanisms underlying these behavioral changes. Just as occurred in victims of early child abuse, the maternally separated pups showed a reduction in their hippocampal volume and alteration in hippocampal morphology. The neurons in the hippocampus had lost many of their dendrites, those little tentacles by which cells in the brain communicate

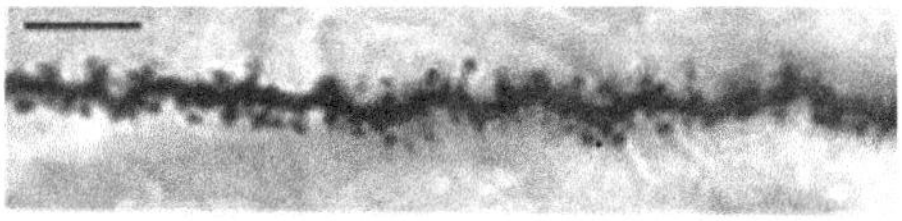

NON-SEPARATED

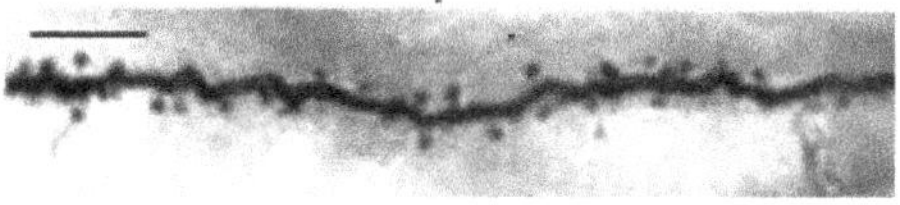

SEPARATED

with each other. There were significant changes also in the amygdala, quite the opposite in fact; there was an increase in volume and cell density with an increase in dendritic branching. As in humans, early life stress in rodents leads to changes in brain anatomy and function, leading to hyperactive responses to all incoming stimuli, including pain; aberrant behaviors are often the result of abnormal sensory processing within the emotional circuitry of the brain. Western medicine has always focused on a peripheral focus for all ailments, but the shift to the inclusion of central mechanisms is the key to understanding most of these medically unexplained disorders.

The "puzzling leap" of Dr. Freud is no longer quite so puzzling or mysterious. We have the neural science to understand how a traumatic childhood translates into long-term molecular and cellular changes that persist throughout life. Psychology IS Biology!!

M. Teicher: Childhood Adversity and Mental Health

G. Tietjen: Childhood Abuse and Migraine Epidemiology, Sex Differences and Potential Mechanisms. HEADACHE. 2011. June; 51 (6): 869-879

Chapter 14

The Reign of Pain is Always in the Brain

Pain figures prominently in many of the medically unexplained disorders, especially the ones that present to medical and specialty clinics. We could not survive without our sensation of pain. One of Descartes's pupils wrote, "God has made man in his own image and likeness, and what better gift could he have given him for his preservation than the sensation of pain?" He developed the famous illustration of "the boy with his foot in the fire".

In this model, pain is envisioned as a one-way path to the brain where it rings the bell. The more potent the stimulus, the louder the bell rings. It is assumed that there is a linear relationship between the strength of the stimulus and the perception of pain. It is a great deal more complex than that, but it is helpful to begin with the analysis of acute pain, where pain equals injury, where hurt equals harm.

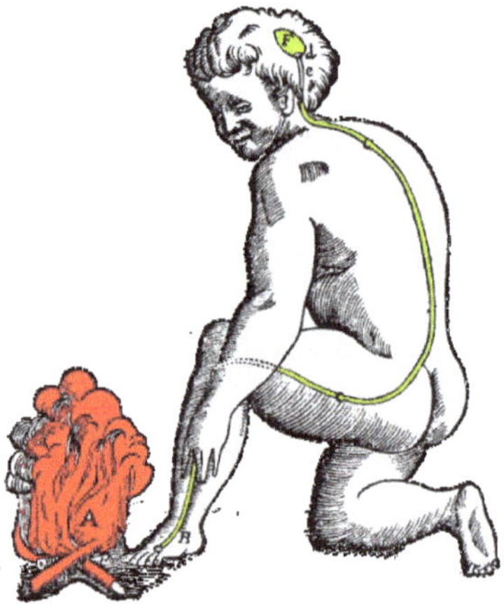

Our brains translate a vast array of signals, both external and internal, into comprehensible sensations. The information contained in an atmospheric compression wave becomes sound. Photons of light are converted into vision. Similarly, mechanical, thermal or chemical assaults on the body are converted into pain signals.

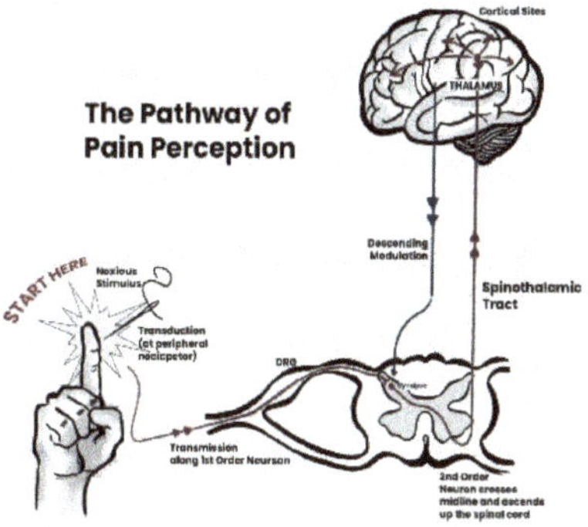

The perception of pain, nociception, starts with *transduction*. This is the process by which noxious stimuli are converted into electrical signals by specialized sensory receptors called nociceptors. These receptors are everywhere in the body except in the brain itself. When tissue damage occurs, from mechanical, thermal or chemical causes, certain chemicals are released which activate the receptors. An electric signal is generated, which is *transmitted* along nerve fibers to the first relay station in the spinal cord, the dorsal horn. At this relay, there is a gate control system that can decrease or increase the strength of the signal. There are two main types of nerve fibers involved in this process, big ones and little ones. The big nerves, A-delta fibers, transmit the pain signal rapidly; the little ones, C-fibers, transmit the dull aching or burning pain that often occurs after the initial pain sensation.

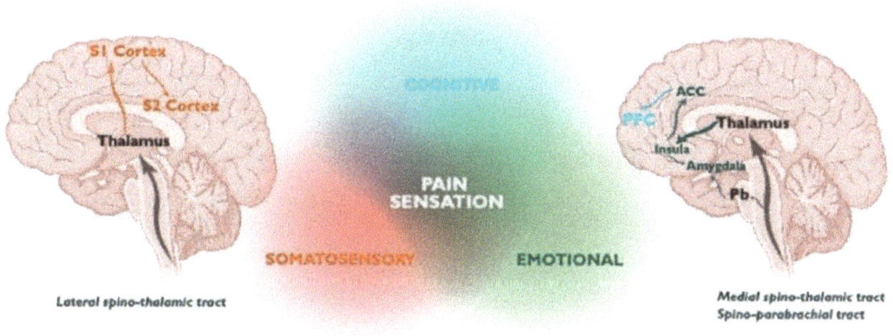

From the spinal cord, the signal is transmitted to higher centers in the brainstem and thalamus, the second great relay station. From the thalamus, the signal splits into a bi-wired system with one division, the lateral pathway, going to the opposite sensory cortex that gives the necessary information about the strength and location of the pain signal. This is the "hurt" or "ouch" part. The other division goes through a more medial pathway into the emotional circuitry of the brain, the limbic system, where the "suffering" or "yuck" part is experienced, and from there to multiple areas in the cortex. Via these neural pathways, multiple brain regions are informed of incoming pain traffic. The brain deciphers the nature and meaning of the pain and responds appropriately, to either amplify or diminish the pain sensation, depending on the needs of the moment. This flexibility is due to the unique nature of the pain system.

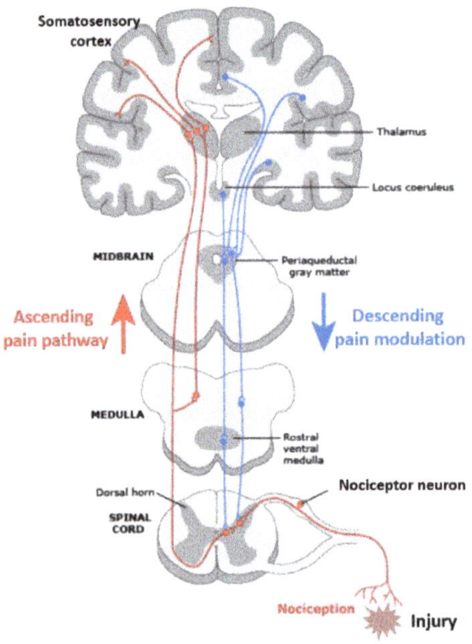

The pain system differs from other sensory systems in that there are two separate systems involved in our perception of pain. One functions as a typical sensory system analogous to other sensory processes. The other is a pain *modulating* system which developed independently of the pain sensory system and actively influences and modulates its functioning. In other words, depending on the nature and the meaning of the pain, the brain responds either by amplifying or diminishing the pain, depending on the needs of the moment. This arrangement allows for maximum flexibility for a behaving organism moving through a dangerous and unpredictable environment. Not surprisingly, the amygdala features prominently in the process. A certain region of the amygdala, the central nucleus, is specific for pain; it is referred to as the nociceptive or pain amygdala. The amygdala is part of the descending pain control system that includes circuits in the brainstem. Thus, the amygdala can modulate pain through descending inhibitory control systems but can also contribute to the generation and enhancement of the pain response. From an evolutionary perspective, it makes sense that the amygdala facilitates pain when pain signals a threat to the body. However, in life-threatening situations when survival is at stake, the amygdala acts to suppress attention to pain. Best not to stop nursing a sprained ankle when running from the saber-toothed tiger.

There is an obvious survival value of pain inhibition in situations of overwhelming stress, but prolonged stress, depression and anxiety may enhance pain. The evolutionary advantages of the former are clear but not so obvious in the latter case, but one fact is obvious, the amygdala is where pain and emotion meet.

The Amygdala in action

In 1946, Lieutenant Colonel Henry K Beecher, an anesthesiologist, published a classic study entitled "The Pain in Men Wounded in Battle". He studied soldiers during prolonged actions in Italy, notably during the assault on the beaches at Anzio. He found that among the most seriously wounded soldiers who were questioned within 12 hours of receiving their wounds, 25% reported only slight pain, 32% reported no pain at all, 75% felt so little pain that in the hours following their wounds, they refused pain medications.

He stated that it was common to see soldiers with hideous injuries report no pain, while the soldier waiting to go into combat would complain loudly of a stubbed toe. Emotions surrounding the event made all the difference; for a soldier, a wound may be a godsend, an honorable way to avoid combat, but for the soldier going into battle, pain is magnified by fear and anxiety.

In civilian life, the same principles apply. The following are two oft-quoted examples of the amygdala at work. In the picture on the left reported in the British Medical Journal in 1995, the following history is reported: This is the case of a builder who jumped down on a 7-inch nail which pierced his boot at toe level. He was in excruciating pain, requiring IV sedation and IV morphine. However, when the boot was cut away, it turned out the nail had fortunately passed between his toes instead of impaling the foot.

In the picture on the right, published in USA Today in 2005, a construction worker unknowingly shot himself in the head with a nail gun and was unaware of the injury. He went to a dentist six days later, complaining of a toothache. Different scenario, different amygdala responses.

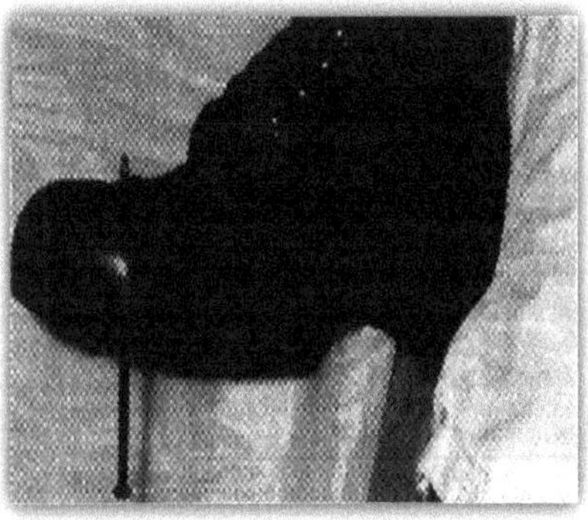

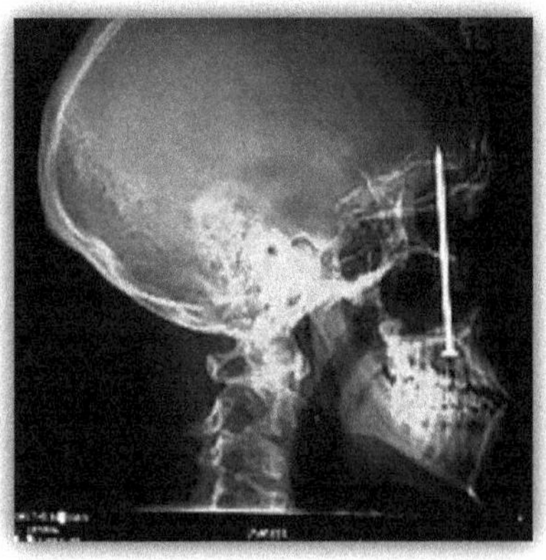

Sensitization: When the Alarm System malfunctions…

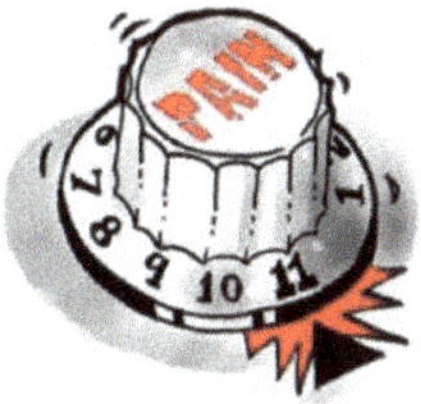

In an ideal world, when the injury is healed, the pain disappears, but there are circumstances where it persists, a meaningless torment serving no biological defensive purpose. The alarm system is just malfunctioning.[34] This phenomenon is called sensitization and can lead to chronic intractable pain regardless of any social, behavioral or psychological factors. If you have ever touched a scalding hot surface, you will know the bright, searing flash of pain. You run to the cold water tap and have immediate but temporary relief. But then comes the after-throb; now the pain is dull, unpleasant, throbbing and sensitive to touch. This hypersensitivity to normally non-painful stimuli is called *allodynia*. This phase is known as peripheral sensitization, and it is a protective adaptive response to avoid further damage to the affected area. There may be hours or days of discomfort, but eventually the tissue heals, and the pain subsides. But, if the pain signal persists, such as happens after an attack of shingles, now the central pathways in the spinal cord and brain begin to change, a process called central sensitization. Repeated pain signals rewire the pain circuitry, leading to a state of hypersensitivity. In these circumstances, pain is no longer a signal of tissue damage; it is a manifestation of a faulty alarm system, like the annoying fire alarm that goes off when you light a candle or the car alarm that shrieks in the night for no good reason other than to disturb your sleep.

Central sensitization features prominently in many disorders such as complex regional pain syndrome (CRPS), "failed back syndrome", phantom limb pain and the burning pain of diabetic neuropathy. These pain disorders, called neuropathic pain disorders, present an enormous challenge. We have a very limited catalog of medications for these disorders, and the usual pain medicines have little effect. The sensitizing process, a device that evolved for our protection, an adaptive strategy, now becomes maladaptive, a major factor in the development of chronic pain syndromes. It is the result of *neural plasticity*, the capacity of neurons in the brain and spinal cord, to change their function and structure.

We spend billions of dollars each year seeking the elusive peripheral pathology when the symptoms are in fact due to altered wiring in the central processing unit of the brain. Yes, the pain is in your head, but not in your imagination.

S. Neugebauer: Amygdala Pain Mechanisms. Nat. Rev. Neuroscience, 16 (7) 920-934

S. Neugebauer: Pain and Emotion: The Crucial Role of the Amygdala. Pain, 130 (1), 1-2. 2007

Wolfe, C.E.: Sensitization: A Critical and Underappreciated Mechanism of Chronic Pain. Pain Medicine, 15 (3), 471-478

Chapter 15
When the Pain is Chronic

Chronic pain features prominently in many medically unexplained disorders and presents the ultimate challenge to modern physicians. In the medical model, a simple algorithm applies: Where there's pain, there's injury, where there's hurt, there's harm. In many chronic pain scenarios, there may be no obvious "harm" as in fibromyalgia and chronic headache. It is very important, however, to remember that many chronic pain disorders begin with obvious peripheral pathology. The pain may continue to persist long after the original lesion or injury has healed and thus transforms itself into a chronic condition that is entirely central and directed by the brain (central sensitization). When the chronic pain disorder begins with obvious pathology, then at least it is a good deal easier to comprehend, if not easier to treat. Pain disorders such as fibromyalgia and chronic headache, where there is no peripheral pathology, are even more challenging.

More of the population is affected by chronic, enduring, life-restricting pain. Like other modern maladies such as drug addiction, alcoholism and obesity, chronic pain is multifactorial with multiple dimensions. There are many on-ramps to the chronic pain highway: age, trauma, diseases, mood disorders, opioid dependency, and chronic stress. It is often difficult to disentangle the contributing factors, but one fact needs to be emphasized: the longer the pain disorder lasts, the more likely that *central* processes are playing a major role.

Chronic pain is not merely acute pain that lasts for a prolonged period, it is a result of rewiring of the pain circuitry in the central nervous system. We should come up with another word for chronic pain and reserve the term "pain" for acute pain. Acute pain follows the "pain = injury model" whereas chronic pain is complex and elusive. Structural changes within the emotional/pain circuits, especially in the amygdala, and the process of sensitization are the key factors in the pathway to chronic pain. The process of sensitization, discussed in the previous chapter, can occur if acute pain is not dealt with effectively. In disorders where nerve pain is predominant, as in shingles or sciatica, the hypersensitivity process can lead to hideous, persistent pain despite our best efforts. These pain disorders do not belong in the "medically unexplained" category; we understand the mechanism whereby this type of pain is generated, even though we lack effective treatments. These pain disorders are associated with mood disorders, but only because of living with chronic pain.

Anxiety and Pain

Many patients with chronic pain exhibit depression and anxiety disorders and many patients with anxiety and depression experience chronic pain, a bidirectional relationship. This should not be surprising since the pain-processing areas of the brain overlap with the systems subserving emotion. For the most part, the emotion is usually negative because pain creates depression and anxiety, and anxiety and depression amplify pain sensations. Anxiety levels have been shown to predict pain severity and pain behavior in both acute and chronic pain patients. It is also well known that anxiety reduction techniques and anxiolytic drugs have been reported to be successful in relieving pain. Virtually no bodily system appears to be unscathed by anxiety. Gastrointestinal illness, respiratory distress, arthritis, metabolic syndromes and musculoskeletal pain all occur at significantly higher rates among people with anxiety disorders. Pain disorders are especially susceptible to negative emotions.

In the course of 50 years of treating patients, especially chronic pain patients, a benzodiazepine has proven to be the most effective option when all else fails. They are not working on "the mind"; they work directly on that portion of the amygdala, the "pain amygdala", which can both amplify and diminish pain sensation. Drugs such as Valium and Ativan have been vilified and demonized in recent years, but used wisely, they are God's gift to the sufferer.

Catastrophizing

"There is nothing good or bad but thinking makes it so."
— Hamlet

Psychologist Michael Sullivan conceives of catastrophizing as "an exaggerated negative mental set brought to bear during actual or *anticipated* pain experience." He has developed a catastrophizing scale; the higher the score, the worse the outcome for the patient. (Remember the construction worker with the nail in his foot that wasn't in his foot).

Medical students are the biggest catastrophizers of all! Sir Arthur Conan Doyle, creator of Sherlock Holmes and himself a physician, dedicated one of his books to:

"The eternal medical student who, during his first close acquaintance with patients and hospital wards, acquires to himself, besides clinical instruction, every disease in the calendar. He first has in his mind that he has tuberculosis of the lungs in a hopeless stage. Endless cigarettes and the smoker's cough help this conviction. Carcinoma of the stomach follows, as a result of late hours and copious draughts of cheap beer. But why does he have sarcoma of the jaw? Elementary, my dear Watson. He is erupting his wisdom teeth!

Obviously a little dated, but I think we get the point. Psychology IS biology.

Burke, N.N.: "Psychological Stress in Early Life as a Predisposing Factor for the Development of Chronic Pain. J. Neurosci. Research. 2017; 95 (6): 1257-1270

Turk, D.: Psychological Factors in Chronic Pain. J. of Consulting and Clinical Psychology. 2002, Vol. 70, No. 3: 678-690

Greden, J.: Depression and Pain. J. Clin. Psychiatry. 69:12. Dec. 2008

Wolfe, C.E.: Sensitization: A Critical and Underappreciated Mechanism of Chronic Pain. Pain Medicine, 15 (3), 471-478

Sullivan, MJL: The Pain Catastrophizing Scale. Psychol. Asses. 1995; 7: 524-32

Chapter 16

Depression and Pain

"If there be a hell upon earth, it is to be found in the melancholy man's heart."
— Robert Burton, The Anatomy of Melancholy (1621)

Depression lurks behind many unexplained disorders both as cause and effect. It has a legacy of disguises and does not always declare itself, at least not to the medical practitioners. In an international study across five continents, 69% of patients with major depression presented with somatic symptoms only. Females presented more bodily symptoms than males. The most frequent symptom among both sexes was pain. These patients haunt pain centers, spinal clinics and headache centers, but they will be grossly insulted and angry if the subject of depression is raised, however, delicately. This is the paradox of depression. It presents not with sadness and tears but with a myriad of physical symptoms.

"James is a 59-year-old accountant with complaints of daily head pressure, dizziness and brain fog. He has seen multiple physicians, had multiple scans, nerve blocks, and medications, but nothing has helped. He lives alone with no intimate partner, but he has maintained an online relationship with a woman in Australia for several months. They chat daily, and she would love to visit, but she needs him to forward the airfare to the US! He has a history of depression, but feels it is no longer a problem.

Family history reveals his father, a military man, was an alcoholic who suffered from depression with several hospitalizations for ECT. Sister died by suicide. He is adamant that he does not feel sad, just exhausted from living with this constant head pressure.

This sad, lonely man is almost certainly suffering from a genetic brain disease. We call it depression, but that name is also used for people experiencing death, loss or disappointment, the slings and arrows of life, "normal depression". James' depression is not a response to loss, and he does not feel sad. This is what is challenging about this condition; it exists on a spectrum, from a predictable reaction to life events to a debilitating brain disorder.

There is no normal Parkinson's disease or normal Multiple Sclerosis. But there is normal depression, and Mother Nature doesn't use a colored marker to indicate transition from normal to pathological. Robert Burton in his 17th-century classic book "The Anatomy of Melancholy" struggled with the difference between normal and abnormal states. He distinguished between melancholy either in disposition or habit,

"There is transitory melancholy which comes and goes upon every small occasion of sorrow, need, sickness, trouble, fear, grief, and passion. Habit is that other melancholy, which is a serious ailment, not errant but fixed, and as it was long increasing, so now grown to a habit, it will hardly be removed. No one has yet improved on this trenchant observation, but there is an urgent need for a more modern diagnostic label for that "other melancholy".

In their 2007 book, "Loss of Sadness", Allan Horwitz and Jerome Wakefield decried the "diseasification" of "normal" sadness but were inevitably vague on the distinction between depressive disorder and normal sadness. It is a deeply personal value judgment as to when sadness ceases to be "proportionate" and becomes a major depressive episode according to DSM 5 criteria. The problem is further compounded by the fact that the range of abnormal is constantly expanding and encroaching on the normal because of the medicalization of culture and the "disease-ifying" of behaviors that are even minimally aberrant.

Can we define brain pathology in depression?

Depression in its extremity is the most intense form of stress. The brain exhibits the same maladaptive changes in depression as it does in prolonged intense stress. It is difficult to pinpoint the exact brain pathology in depression, but not surprisingly, the hippocampus and amygdala feature prominently. The hippocampus appears to be especially vulnerable. It is one of the few brain regions to undergo neurogenesis (producing new brain cells), which is vital to its role in memory formation. Shrinkage of the hippocampus was one of the first brain changes observed in depression, which may account for the "pseudodementia" seen in severe depression.

A recent report in **Science** vol. 391, 2026, highlights the changes in the brain with pain and depression. In patients and in an animal model, early stages of chronic pain were found to be associated with an increase in hippocampal volume, whereas later stages were associated with decreased hippocampal volume. These changes in rats were followed by the development of depressive-like behavior. The authors showed that activation of microglial cells, which are typically scavenger cells, leads to impaired hippocampal neurogenesis (growth of new cells) with diminished volume, and shifts in hippocampal physiology leading to depressive behavior. This is clear proof that depression and chronic pain are two sides of the same neurobiological coin.

The amygdala shows increased activity and enlargement. Functional neuroimaging studies have constantly shown that the amygdala becomes more reactive to emotional and other stimuli in major depression.

Changes also occur in the pre-frontal cortex, PFC, with decreased volume and decreased activity, which lead to cognitive impairment and emotional dysregulation.

This is the perfect storm, a weakened cortex and hippocampus (which moderate amygdala activity) and an enlarged, hyperactive amygdala, which amplifies all incoming sensory stimuli: Non-painful stimuli transformed into pain and painful stimuli magnified. No mysterious alchemy, just a faulty central processor as in Michael Meaney's rats.

There is another neurophysiological reason why depression is painful. There are inhibitory pathways descending from the brain to the spinal cord, which provide a mechanism whereby pain is modified or even eliminated. These descending pathways are fueled by the same neurotransmitters that are implicated in depression. When these neurotransmitters are depleted, then the pain inhibitory system is also affected. Pain and depression are Siamese twins, pain leading to depression and depression leading to pain.

Treatment

For most of the last century, depression was viewed as a purely psychological disorder. In recent decades, the "chemical imbalance" theory has prevailed with a profusion of drug treatments. A recent report from the British newspaper, The Observer, notes that Prozac is now detected in the drinking water in Great Britain. More than any other human disorder, depression eludes any simplistic explanation or tidy neurochemical theory. For decades, we have relied on the serotonin deficiency syndrome as the basis for depression, anxiety and OCD, but recently this theory has come under heavy fire. In 2022 and 2023, **Molecular Psychiatry** published a landmark "umbrella review" that fundamentally challenged the long-standing serotonin hypothesis of depression. The central study, led by Joanna Moncrieff and colleagues, synthesized decades of research across six major areas to evaluate whether depression is caused by low serotonin levels. Their primary conclusion was that there was no convincing evidence that depression is associated with, or caused by, lower serotonin concentrations or activity. (Another example of the "tragedy of Science", a beautiful theory destroyed by ugly fact…Thomas Huxley). But do not despair, the authors have given us a new theory of depression:

"According to the current state of evidence-based knowledge, depression represents a dysbalanced dynamic system involving genetic, epigenetic, environmental and stress vulnerabilities initiating a cascade of neurobiological alterations in and beyond the serotonergic functioning. These alterations are reflected by

impaired neurotransmission, attenuated neuroplasticity and neurogenesis, dysfunctional neural circuitries, hypothalamic-pituitary axis (HPA) abnormalities, increased inflammation and vascular changes, whereby monoamines, including serotonin, norepinephrine, and dopamine, as well as glutamate, GABA, glucocorticoids, inflammatory cytokines and neurotrophic factors, including the brain-derived neurotrophic factor, seemed to be essential mediators."(This is certainly an all-embracing theory, but one that will take some time to unpack and its immediate relevance to the clinician is not readily apparent)

So now that the serotonin deficiency idea has been debunked, the question arises, why have we been pushing drugs that elevate the serotonin level if, in fact, there never has been a serotonin deficiency? For years, we freely dispensed antidepressant drugs, confident that we were correcting a neurochemical deficiency, when we were very likely administering a placebo, at least in many cases.

Several years ago, Irving Kirsch, director of the Program in Placebo Studies and lecturer in medicine at Harvard Medical School, generated a great deal of controversy by questioning the therapeutic benefits of antidepressant drugs. He wrote, "analysis of the published and the unpublished clinical trial data are consistent in showing that most, if not all, of the benefits of antidepressants in the treatment of depression and anxiety are due to the placebo response, and the difference in improvement between drug and placebo is not clinically meaningful".

More than 30 million Americans now take antidepressants, which would be acceptable if they actually worked, but recent analysis shows that the gap between active drug and placebo has shrunk to the point that antidepressant drugs are essentially placebos. Psychedelic-based medications hold great promise for the future. Many studies are underway and it is likely that psychedelic-assisted therapy will soon be approved for depression, anxiety disorders, OCD, and addiction.

The whole situation is downright depressing! We cannot really define what depression is, we cannot identify the pathophysiological basis, and we don't have any truly effective medicines. It is a very sneaky disorder with an endless supply of guises, confounding patients and physicians alike. In almost every medically unexplained disorder, it is there but must be extracted from the presenting symptoms with some caution. It is a challenge to raise the issue with a patient who comes with physical symptoms. They have already converted their "unease" into disease and are expecting a medical solution. They think depression is "feeling sad" but will protest firmly, I'm not depressed, I hurt!

Every once in a while, we are gifted with a clear, unambiguous cause for depression:

Mary Ellen was in her mid-60s, mother of fifteen children, who managed her complicated and demanding children with enormous patience and love, the latter dished out in barely manageable portions. She never complained and always seemed to be singing some tuneless melody as she baked bread or scrubbed the linoleum floor. Her children venerated her and vied for her attention. Then, without warning, the seeming solidity of their world fell apart. Mother no longer rose out of bed in the morning to stoke the fire and bake the bread. She turned her face to the wall and refused food. Doctor O' Dwyer was summoned and his arrival with that iconic black bag always seemed to cure everything. The good doctor was mystified but did leave a "bottle" to be administered daily. The bottle had no effect other than to force her to go to the toilet multiple times. Even the priest was called for, but Mary Ellen, never the overly religious type, listened politely and turned her face to the wall as soon as he left. In the night, the children heard a sound they had never heard before, their mother weeping. And then, the cure! She arose from the bed one day to announce that it was the "bloody pill" that was making her sick. The bloody pill was Rautrax, a blood pressure medicine that contains the active ingredient reserpine. Reserpine depletes the stores of vital neurotransmitters, those chemicals vital for communication between brain cells. It's major side-effect? Depression. Within a week of stopping the drug, we could hear her tra la la while scrubbing the floor. Our mother was back! To paraphrase Samuel Johnson, "thus I refute Moncrieff."

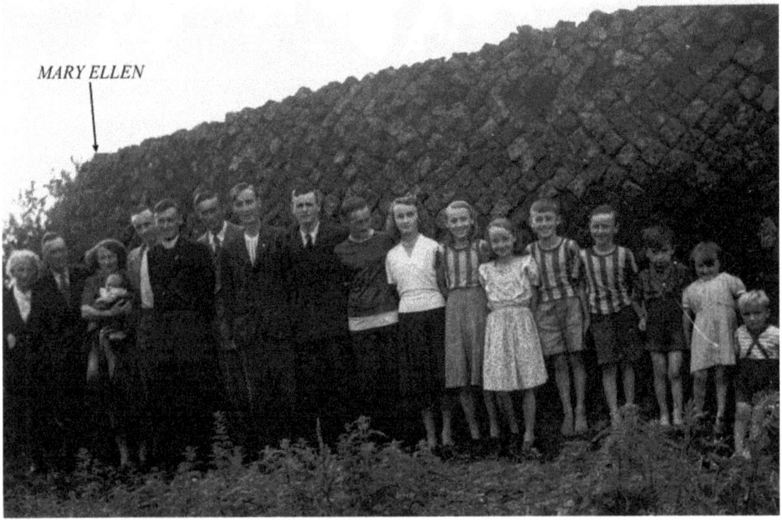

By now, it should be clear that chronic pain disorders are multifaceted and do not conform to the "pain equals injury" model. Regardless of the mechanisms involved, chronic pain is a central processing disorder. If most chronic pain is central, then it does not require nerve blocks and operations that affect the peripheral pathways, but doctors cling to a peripheralist model that often leads to useless, expensive and invasive treatment of chronic pain. Most physicians are dogged peripheralists, not merely because of financial gain but because our training for over a century has taught us nothing else.

Katon, W.J. (2001) "Epidemiology and Treatment of Depression in Chronic Pain Settings. Psych Clinics of North America, 24 (4) 557-570
Thompson, L.G. (2016): The Relationship Between Depression and Chronic Pain: A Review. Journal of Clinical Psychology, 72 (1) 16-30
Horwitz, Allan V., Wakefield, Jerome C. The Loss of Sadness. Oxford University Press. 2007.

Chapter 17
Placebo

"The history of medical treatment is essentially the history of the placebo effect."
— Anne Harrington, Professor of the History of Medicine, Harvard University

Yet another example of the neural plasticity of the pain pathways is the phenomenon of placebo. This is the phenomenon where patients experience improvements in their condition after receiving a substance or treatment that has no therapeutic effect. Placebos can take various forms, such as sugar pills, saline injections or even sham surgeries. All of these "treatments" are designed to mimic the appearance of the actual treatment without containing any active ingredients. Until the 1940's and the arrival of penicillin, doctors had little to offer. Throughout the ages, patients submitted to purging, puking, poisoning, cutting, cupping, bleeding, leeching and shocking and the physicians were respected, honored and paid, even though these "treatments" did more harm than good.

In the 19th and early 20th century, there was a thriving market for patent medicines and homeopathic cures. As late as the 1950's, general practitioners in Britain were dispensing a placebo to 40% of their patients. A major factor in the efficacy of placebo was some dramatic effect, therapeutic or not. Purgatives were a favorite: after multiple trips to the toilet, the patient always knew they had been "dosed."

Then, in the late 1970's, there was a much-heralded discovery of certain naturally occurring substances in the brain called endorphins. They are similar to opium-derived pain killers and attach themselves to the same receptor sites in the brain as morphine. Levine and Fields administered saline or water to college students following dental surgery. The students showed marked improvement, which was predictable enough, but then they administered naloxone, a drug that blocks the effects of morphine and other opioids. The placebo effects were reversed, demonstrating that placebo works by releasing our own morphine-like substance, the endorphins.

Placebo also works in reverse, it's called Nocebo. Eighty percent of hospitalized patients were given sugar water and told that it was an emetic, a drug to produce vomiting, subsequently vomited. Expectation was crucial to the outcome. The same principle applies to animals.

In 1975, Robert Ader and colleagues were studying taste-aversion in rats. Rats love saccharin-flavored water and lap it up when presented. In the study, saccharin-flavored water was paired with injections of cyclophosphamide, a nausea-inducing drug. The researchers had not realized that cyclophosphamide is a powerful immunosuppressant agent used to treat cancer. Predictably, the rats became sick, and some died. A sub-group of rats continued to be fed drinks of saccharin water without the injections, but they continued to die at high rates. It seemed that the saccharin drink, originally associated by the rats with the injections, now triggered the same powerful immunosuppressant effects as the cyclophosphamide itself. Later, Ader said, "I had no idea that the brain was connected to the immune system."

The placebo effect even applies to surgical procedures. Sham surgery is now approved for clinical trials. Sham surgery or placebo surgery is a faked surgical intervention that omits the step thought to be therapeutically necessary. In many minimally invasive surgical procedures and injection treatments, the sham procedure was as good as the real operation.

It is fair to say that placebo is as effective a pain medicine as any of the more expensive products on the market. The same is true for psychiatric medications. Pharmaceutical companies have essentially given up on developing new antidepressant medications since it is becoming more difficult to extract a real therapeutic benefit for the new drug. In the clinical trials, the placebo was almost as effective as the study drug. The much-revered Galen knew the value of placebo: "He cures most successfully in whom the patient has most confidence."

It is important to point out, however, that the placebo effect applies in situations where there are subjective outcomes such as pain and depression. Placebo has no such impact on cancer.

Anne Harrington. The Cure Within. Norton 2008.
J D Levine, N C Gordon, H L Fields, Lancet. 1978 Sep 23;2 (8091): 654-7
Richard Kradin. The Placebo Response. Routledge 2008
Ader, R. Psychosomatic and psychoimmunologic research. Psychosomatic Medicine, 42,307-321 1980

Chapter 18

Fibromyalgia: The Queen of Medically Unexplained Disorders

Jane is a 56-year-old executive who presents with diffuse musculoskeletal pain, fatigue and insomnia. She reported that these symptoms began several years ago without any obvious cause. She admits that her job is especially stressful but denies that it is playing any role in her symptoms. She admits to being verbally and emotionally abused by a domineering, alcoholic father. "Nothing I did was ever good enough." Mother suffered from depression and chronic anxiety. Jane is twice divorced, both ex-husbands are also alcoholics. She has one adult daughter with whom she has a difficult relationship.

She brought a large, beautifully organized binder containing her extensive medical history, which included chronic headache, irritable bowel disorder and "mast-cell disorder". She feels that all of her symptoms are caused by "inflammation" and "autoimmune," but her rheumatologist feels that fibromyalgia is the main cause of her symptoms. She is currently disabled because of debilitating fatigue and pain and requests that I sign a form supporting her disability claim.

Clinically well-defined medical disorders do not provoke controversy, but in the case of fibromyalgia, there is heated debate as to its validity as a real medical disease. Like other chronic MUDs, there is no biomarker, no obvious physical findings and all lab tests are negative. There are only symptoms and no signs. Doctors have long debated the nature of this modern malady; they are divided into believers and non-believers. Dr. Frederick Wolfe, a true believer and proselytizer for fibromyalgia as a medical disease, subsequently wrote:

"Perhaps selecting tender points as the essential criteria for defining FM was a mistake. By ignoring the central psychosocial

and distress features of the syndrome and choosing instead a physical examination item, we allowed FM to be seen mostly as a physical illness."

Most reasonable physicians would agree with Dr. Wolfe that fibromyalgia is not a classical disease while acknowledging its multifactorial nature and its impact on patients' lives. In this disorder, as in other nebulous "disease of the month" conditions, patients are active collaborators in the medicalization of their problems. But this disorder cannot be dismissed as a cultural artifact. It is not a classical disease, but it is still a product of the brain / mind (braind) and deserves our respect and compassion.

Women and Pain

Kristin K. Barker in her book, Fibromyalgia, 2005, writes: *"After more than two decades of committed research, the biomedical understanding of fibromyalgia syndrome FMS, is still tenuous and highly contentious. There are no objective indicators of the disorder, nor are there clear theoretical accounts for what causes the disorder. There is disagreement about its pathogenic characteristics and there are no genuinely effective treatment options. The almost total absence of sex or gender from the framing of FMS, therefore, is all the more peculiar, given that perhaps the only uncontested fact about this highly contested disorder is its feminization."*

Skeptics say that fibromyalgia is medicalized unhappiness, and that doctors and big pharma are creating pseudo-diseases. While it is certain that social, cultural and psychological factors play a major role, *the most glaringly obvious feature of this disorder and indeed of all the medically unexplained disorders, is the preponderance of female sufferers. There are many dimensions to the medicalization* of women's bodily complaints, involving sex (biology) and gender (culture)

Is FM just the newest manifestation of that ancient malady, hysteria? Towards the end of the 19th century, doctors diagnosed complaints of females as "Neurasthenia", a chronic fatigue syndrome first identified by George Beard, 1839-1883, the American neurologist. It was also known as "American Nervousness" or "Nervous Exhaustion," (a term still favored by rock stars entering drug rehab!) He considered the condition to be an organic nervous disorder triggered by excess intellectual, sexual or digestive activity. He wrote, "the symptoms are dyspepsia, headaches, insomnia, paresthesias, weakness, neuralgia, rheumatism, wet dreams and painful periods".

Neurasthenia was enthusiastically received at home and abroad. *"Since the works of George Beard, a new nervous disease has been imported from America and seems to be propagated like an epidemic. The name of Neurasthenia is on everybody's lips; It is the fashionable new disease,"* Paul Dubois, Paris, 1904.

As the florid manifestations of hysteria gradually receded in the 20th century, they were replaced by fatigue and pain. Feminist historians view fibromyalgia as a culturally determined and societally sanctioned style of somatization, feelings of frustration and anger at the constraints of the patriarchy, converting into physical symptoms. If you swallow rage, you get indigestion!

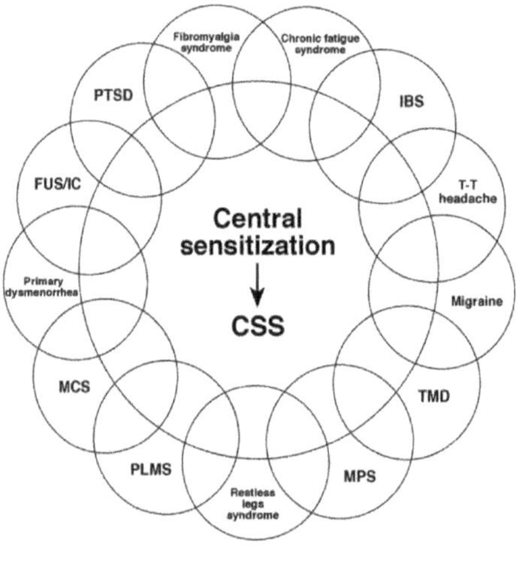

YUNUS, 2000

Not one medical treatise, book or paper, has ever addressed this issue. Female novelists and sociologists have been writing about this glaring omission for the last century, but the medical model simply ignores it. It is a complicated matter, to be sure, but it is time for the male-dominated medical profession to address it. There has been an influx of females into the profession in the last century, but they are surprisingly silent about this and other female concerns, such as the neurobiology of menopause. It is now accepted that FM is mostly a central processing disorder, or as it is often called, a *central sensitivity disorder (CSS) Yunus*. Like many other MUDs, there are shared characteristics. Childhood abuse, anxiety and depression are prominent in this population. Approximately 70% of fibromyalgia patients have depression and studies demonstrate that mood disorders predate the onset of FM in most cases. How adverse experience is converted into symptoms is no longer a mystery. Alterations in the emotional and pain-processing pathways create a heightened sensitivity to painful and even non-painful stimuli. This is the core pathophysiology of this and other central sensitivity disorders. Psychology IS Biology.

In a 2000 paper (Pain Med, March 2000) Rome and Rome introduced the concept of limbically augmented pain syndrome (LAPS). It offered a neurobiological basis for the effect of mood and stress on pain perception. They speculated that aberrations in the limbic structure, especially the amygdala, led to heightened perception of pain. The concepts of LAPS and CSS are integrative theories uniting mind and brain.

Yunus, M.: Fibromyalgia and Overlapping Disorders: The Unifying Concept of Central Sensitivity Syndrome. Semin. Arthritis Rheum. 36: 339-356

Sluka / Clauw: Neurobiology of Fibromyalgia and Chronic Widespread Pain. Neuroscience 2016, Dec. 3; 338: 114 - 129.

Chapter 19
Headache

"If you want to show someone the difficulties of medical practice, give them a headache patient."
— Oliver Wendell Holmes

If fibromyalgia is the queen of MUDs, then headache is the lady-in-waiting. If fibromyalgia is a feminized disorder, so is headache. The overwhelming majority of patients who consult a neurologist for headaches are female. For thousands of years, it has been identified as a uniquely female disorder and therefore stigmatized, as just a "female problem". That stigma still lingers. Despite its epidemic proportions, the average medical student gets minimal, if any, instructions on how to manage the headache patient. It does not conform to the medical model of disease and is frequently affected by that messy stuff called life.

In the course of 14 years of training, medical school, internal medicine residency, neurology residency, and fellowship, there was no education on the topic of headache. There was never a brain-cutting conference devoted to headache! Yet when I entered practice, I was assailed by headache patients. It took time to realize that headache disorders did not behave according to the medical model. The longer the disorder lasts, the more likely it is that stress, mood, and behavior play a major role. I was often frustrated since the factors contributing to their disorder were often outside of my power to help. There have been many occasions in the past where I have tried everything to help an unfortunate headache sufferer, only to have them return to my office, with a new complaint, but headache-free. The solution? Ending an unhappy marriage. Even more frustrating were the patients who went to an alternative practitioner, a chiropractor or acupuncturist and got better. How dare they! (It takes a few years and some life lessons to get over the hubris of the freshly minted doctor).

There are over 300 different causes of headaches, but migraine is the default diagnosis when confronted by a headache patient. For the purposes of this book, headache means migraine.

Migraine

Migraine is a recurrent, genetic, neurovascular disorder. It is the ideal disorder to slice through the mind-body dilemma: it is a biological disorder, whose "creds" are well established, but one which is profoundly influenced by emotional and behavioral factors. ("Every migraine is drenched with emotion", Oliver Sachs). Migraine begins in the brain, but the pain of migraine occurs outside the brain, in the meninges (the membranes which line the brain) and blood vessels of the scalp. Virtually all of the research in the last few decades has focused on the pain of migraine, but we have progressed very little in understanding the actual brain component. For most patients, pain is their greatest concern, and there has been tremendous success in understanding and treating the pain of migraine. Yet the brain stuff remains a mystery, with a variety of neurological symptoms, visual aura, vertigo, numbness, weakness and speech disturbance. Other organ systems are also affected, cardiac and especially gastrointestinal. Migraine is more than a headache!

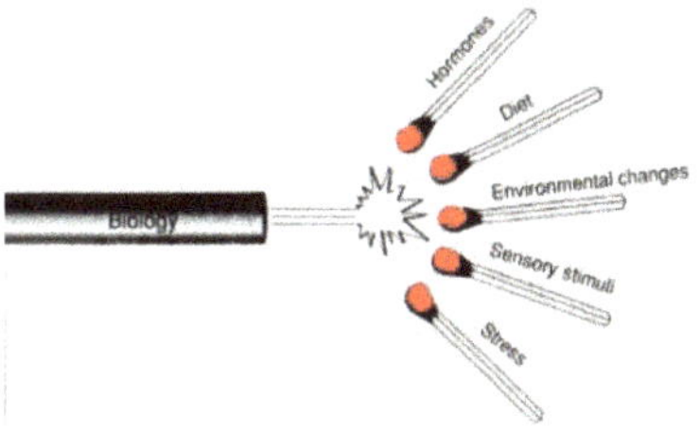

While migraine is a genetic disorder, it can be activated by a huge variety of triggers. Hormonal fluctuations in females are a major trigger, but external stimuli such as light, sound, smell, altitude and even atmospheric fluctuations can all play a role. Stress is a key factor for many patients. Migraine has been dubbed the other IBS, the "irritable brain syndrome". (Some speculate that a hypervigilant, hyperresponsive nervous system may have had a survival value for a hunter-gatherer, but it is very clear that it has outlived its usefulness for modern humans.)

Migraine exists on a *spectrum*, from an intermittent, easily manageable disorder to chronic, relentless misery. There is an enormous difference between a young woman who is afflicted with a menstrual-related migraine headache once every couple of months and a patient who comes with a 20-year history of daily headache. Physicians can easily manage the digestible part of the spectrum, but struggle when it comes to dealing with the other end, where the disorder has become chronic, resistant to treatment and associated with mood disorders and chronic stress. These are the 2-4 % of chronic headache sufferers who haunt the emergency rooms (where they are often dubbed "frequent flyers") and headache clinics. This is MUD territory!

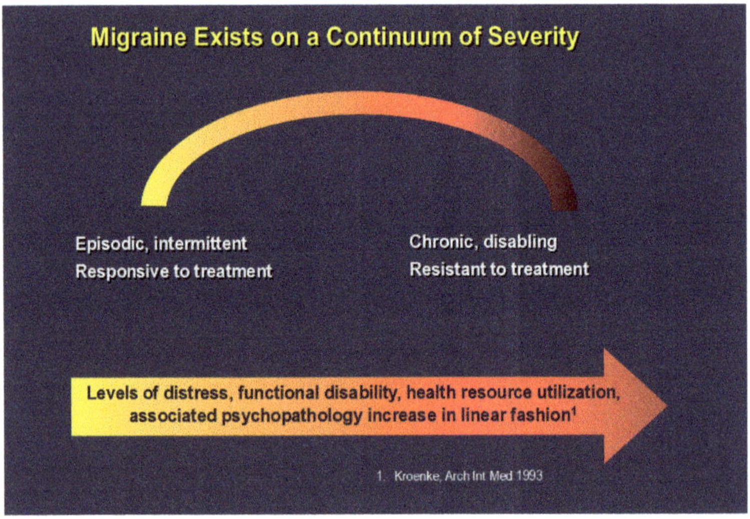

Chronic Migraine: The 2-4%

Intermittent migraine attacks are easy to treat, given the multitude of effective medications now readily available. A young migraine sufferer with an occasional monthly menstrual migraine does not need a psychologist; she needs medicine, but the chronic sufferer presents a unique challenge. The pathway to the chronic end of the spectrum is depressingly familiar. Over 85% of patients with chronic migraine have a history of childhood trauma, neglect and abandonment. Most chronic headache sufferers are women, another "feminized" disorder. This is the primary reason why migraine is *stigmatized* as "just a female problem". There are also coexisting disorders, mostly irritable bowel syndrome, fibromyalgia, insomnia, chronic fatigue, brain fog, and depression. It's all biological, but biology has been hijacked by stress, either childhood or current. Mood disorders, depression and anxiety play a major role. The chronic migraine sufferer is subjected to an incredible variety of investigations and treatments: their eyes are refracted, the TMJ's are adjusted, allergies are desensitized, sinus cavities excavated, recurrent courses of antibiotics for non-existent sinus infections, epidural steroid injections and nerve blocks, necks chiropracted, and finally, the coup de grâce, cervical laminectomy and fusion. But wait, there's more! Of late, the plastic surgeons have entered the fray. They just free up those nerves and remove troublesome muscles, all for a staggering fee! Of all the chronic pain disorders, the migraine sufferer is the most abused, which is a sad irony, since many sufferers, almost all female, have a history of childhood abuse.

Doctors and especially neurologists often resist any psychological or behavioral interpretations as if such associations undermine the biological and scientific nature of the disorder. They constantly emphasize that migraine is a "real disease", an assertion supported by pharmaceutical companies who are equally invested in the disease model. (As a life-long migraine sufferer, I reject the disease label. I prefer to call it a "disorder", one that I share with millions of human beings across the globe.) Adding insult to injury, migraine is constantly misdiagnosed, thus missing the opportunity to treat it in its intermittent, manageable state. By the time the chronic migraine patient seeks help, it has become a central processing disorder.

There are other on-ramps to the chronic headache highway, happy childhood or no.

Martha is a 71-year-old retired physicist who had been a migraine sufferer for much of her life, but only occasionally and responsive to medication. Then she began to experience daily debilitating headaches. She could not identify any specific cause but brought with her an array of MRI scans of the head and neck, all of which were normal. She wanted one more saying, "there's something wrong and no one is able to find it". With a little patience I was able to discover that the escalation began 23 1/2 months prior. (She is a physicist and very precise). When asked about the significance of that date, she stated, "That is when Luigi died". Martha was unmarried, had no children, had spent most of her life at MIT so I assumed that Luigi was a much-loved pet. She wept through a box of Kleenex before asking if I would like to see a picture of Luigi. I agreed, imagining that I would see an adorable dog or cat, but Luigi was a goldfish! I also noticed a large, embossed certificate behind Luigi, which was an actual baptismal certificate. She had taken Luigi in a portable aquarium to a weekend retreat sponsored by a local order of monks. (The retreat was for her.) A very understanding friar baptized Luigi at her request.

What to do? Relying on my extensive academic training, I came up with a novel treatment: she had to go immediately and purchase another goldfish. She hesitated, worried that it might be a "betrayal of Luigi's memory", but I insisted and carried the day. Now she drops by periodically, not for any medical problem, her headache long since resolved, but to present me with some obscure paper on quantum mechanics after I had professed an interest in that topic. I do not know which is more mysterious, quantum mechanics or the workings of the human mind. Sadly, despite all the consultations and scans, no one had asked this solitary woman about her life or the significance of the timing of the onset of her headache. Her diagnosis from her headache specialist, "New Daily Persistent Headache, NDPH." I have never encountered such a disorder without a cause, it just takes time and persistence to discover it.

Mood and Migraine

There are other pathways to the chronic migraine highway, which is essentially another *chronic pain disorder*. As expected, depression is a major factor both as a cause and effect. There is a fivefold greater incidence of major depression in the chronic migraine population. It is rare to encounter a chronic headache patient who is not on an antidepressant or who does not have a family history of depression.

These patients are anxious and prone to catastrophizing. I know of no other human malady that lends itself to catastrophizing as much as this recurrent, unpredictable disorder. The unfortunate sufferer is either recovering from an attack, in the grips of one or dreading the next one. This often leads to an ever- increasing dependency on medications and "medication-overuse-headache", (MOH), which serves only to increase the frequency and intensity of the attacks through some hitherto unknown mechanism. With repeated attacks, the phenomenon of sensitization takes place, shifting the action from pain receptors in the scalp and blood vessels to central pathways in the brain. In fact, pain pathways in the brain become so sensitized that the slightest provocation, missing a meal, sleeping in late on a Saturday morning or a quarrel with one's spouse, can trigger an attack.

Behavioral Factors in Chronic Migraine

Not all patients with chronic headache and other medically mysterious disorders are victims of abuse or neglect. Social learning plays a role. There is another factor to consider. Migraine is not a fatal disorder. It lasts a lifetime, enough time to become encrusted with behavioral issues. Fatal diseases are rarely so burdened for obvious reasons. Chronic disorders become part of our behavioral repertoire. "Not tonight dear, I have a headache", is an enduring trope, but pain is a remarkably adaptable and useful standby if one wishes to avoid an unpleasant situation. After years of chronic migraine, the pattern becomes embedded in the nervous system, a default response to life stress. It is important to point out that not all patients with chronic headache and other medically mysterious disorders are victims of abuse or neglect. Social learning plays a role. Symptoms can become chronic as a consequence of learning from parental reactions to their symptoms. Young patients are especially vulnerable. It is very common to see a young migraine sufferer accompanied by the "helicopter" parent who is constantly obsessing about their pain. Pain becomes the language of communication, and it is a delicate task to extricate the child from smothering mothering. Chronic illness, real or imagined, involves family, friends, caregivers and employers. Alterations in brain anatomy are not the only, nor the primary, factors involved in the development of chronic headache and other medically unexplained disorders. Sometimes illness is a way of being, especially when sickness behavior is so rewarded.

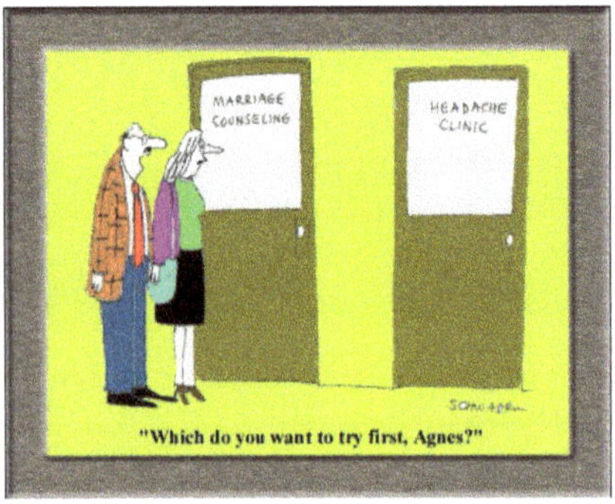

Professor M is in his 80s but still practicing as a pathologist at a local hospital. On every visit, he is accompanied by his wife, who keeps a meticulous record of his daily struggle with headache. She has been monitoring his headache disorder for over 50 years and has kept a scroll with a timeline highlighting the various treatments, all of which have failed. She unravels the document which now is beginning to look like the Dead Sea Scrolls. She is the one who relates his symptoms and the various triggers for his pain. The professor sits quietly, allowing his wife to be his spokesperson. She monitors all food and drink and brings his lunch to his office every day. Mrs. M is fond of saying, "My husband is a martyr," to which the professor modestly bends his head in acquiescence. My contribution is merely to reinforce his martyr-like status and acknowledge the failure of our medicines. Both seem quite satisfied by this admission and return every 3 months so that Mrs. M can update me on his struggle.

It would be a very foolish physician who would attempt to interfere in this longstanding mode of being, the professor as victim, his wife as savior. Withdraw with humility from the field and save your energy for the next battle. Dr. Harold Wolff, the "father" of headache medicine in the US, stated, *"the decision to relinquish a headache disorder is ultimately in the hands of the patient; they must choose to embrace the possibility of change and take an active role in their own healing."* This observation applies to many of the medically unexplained disorders where personal choice plays a role in the return to health. This is an alien concept to physicians, who view themselves as the sole agents in the healing process.

Buse, D.C. (2012): "The Effects of Life-Style Factors on Migraine: A Review". Current Pain and Headache Reports, 16 (3), 220 – 229.
Ashina, M. (2020): "Behavioral and Psychological Aspects of Migraine". Current Opinion in Neurology, 33 (3) 351 – 356.
Suzuki, K. Central Sensitization in Migraine. J. Pain Research. 7 Sept. 2022.

Chapter 20

Chronic Fatigue Syndrome (CFS)

Chronic fatigue syndrome was known as the malaise of the 80s and then the medical syndrome of the 90s, known as "tired all the time or TATT." The official handbook of the American Patient Network describes it as follows: "CFS rips apart the lives of its victims, often incapacitating them in the prime of life while shattering personal relationships and destroying careers. The illness is causing alarm within the scientific community and hardship and heartbreak among the afflicted".

For those of us who deal with devastating neurologic diseases such as Alzheimer's or Lou Gehrig's disease, this may sound like hyperbole, but we must respect its reality and its impact on patients' lives. Patients with chronic fatigue are still viewed with suspicion and derision by the medical culture that looks down on "psychogenic" illness. Patients seek validation from "alternative" practitioners who ply them with proprietary supplements, heavy metal detox and colonic irrigation and hyperbaric oxygen chambers.

Ellen is a 53-year-old woman with a long history of chronic fatigue, brain fog and fibromyalgia. She has a history of recurrent depressive episodes and has been on numerous psychotropic medications, but with only transient benefit. She is a professor at a local college, married but not happily. She has one child, a son, who has been in rehab several times. I did what every physician should do, empathize and validate. I spent quite some time explaining the brain-body connection in an effort to destigmatize the "psych part." By this time, she was on disability as a result of the debilitating fatigue. Many months later, she returned to tell me that she had been diagnosed with Chronic Lyme. The specialist in question placed her on multiple supplements and vitamins, which are costing her a fortune, but she was very grateful that she finally knew the cause of her misery. (Once disability becomes a factor, the chances of any significant treatment are slim and none.)

Like other MUDs, these symptoms are subjective and cannot be proven or disproven. It has often been attributed to a viral illness. In 1984, following the identification of the Epstein-Barr virus and its popularization by the press, there was a virtual epidemic of flu-like illness and fatigue. In New York magazine, writer Steve Pond warned that "a mysterious epidemic is sweeping Hollywood. Screenwriters, actors, producers and studio executives alike are coming down with Epstein Barr, a nonfatal viral syndrome that causes deep fatigue and has no known cure". Many of the patients in the early years of the "epidemic" were young professionals, including athletes, executives and musicians, leading to the nickname "yuppie flu", the malaise of Young Urban Professionals. Multiple factors were implicated, including over-exertion and stress; in Scandinavia, leakage from dental amalgam was implicated. But in the US, the viral theory has remained popular.

Chronic fatigue syndrome is often coupled with Myalgic Encephalomyelitis (ME), which sounds very "medical", even fatal, but of course it is no more fatal than CFS. (It is somewhat ironic that the acronym ME suggests the self-absorption of these patients rather than the lethality of the disorder). Simon Wessely, a psychiatrist who has written extensively on this and other MUDs, points out that 90% of CFS patients are white and female. He states, with perhaps a touch of irony, that "it seems not to be diagnosed among ethnic minorities".

It is easy to be cynical about such phenomena, but it reflects broader issues with medically unexplained symptoms: It shows how cultural factors shaped our understanding of illness, particularly ones that resist easy biological explanation. The failure of the medical model to address these disorders has created a vacuum filled by what Elizabeth Egan, writing in the NYT, calls the "Wellness-Industrial complex", now a $5.6 trillion global industry. This industry exists because the medical profession is still mired in the 19th century.

ME/CFS Basics. CDC. May 10, 2024

Chapter 21

Irritable Bowel Syndrome (IBS)

Mind and Gut

- Scared shitless
- Swallow frustration
- Bad taste in our mouth
- Butterflies in our stomach
- Gut feeling
- Gut-wrenching
- Gut reaction
- Sick to my stomach
- Knots in my stomach

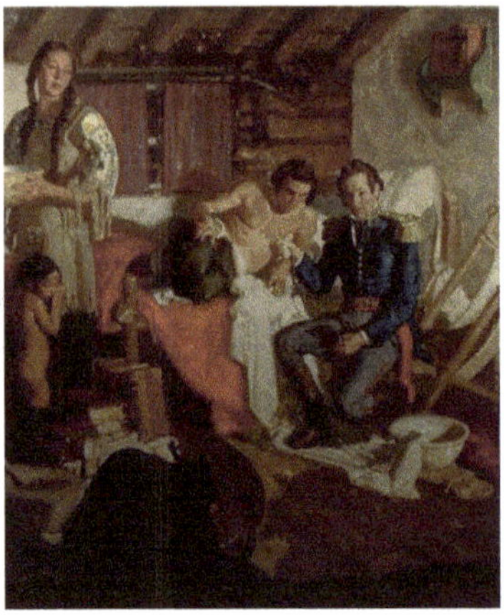

DR WILLIAM BEAUMONT AND THE UNFORTUNATE ALEXIS ST MARTIN

Experiments and Observations on the Gastric Juice and Physiology of Digestion 1833

In 1822, an unfortunate fellow called Alexis St. Martin sustained a gunshot wound to the chest during an altercation with a fellow drinker. He was left with a large open wound, allowing access to his stomach. William Beaumont, an army surgeon often referred to as the father of gastric physiology, took this opportunity to study the effects of emotion on the digestive process. He made many momentous discoveries on the nature of digestion, but he also observed the influence of mental disturbance on the secretion of gastric juice and the digestive process. St. Martin's digestion slowed when he felt irritable and depressed. If Phineas Gage showed that the body affects mind, Alexis St. Martin showed that the mind/brain affects the body, that the mental affects the physical. Beaumont's work contributed to the understanding of the mind/brain-body connection, illustrating how psychological factors could influence physiological processes. (Subsequently, Beaumont was criticized for failing to treat Alexis, whom he could have easily cured; instead, he merely observed him as one would a laboratory animal.)

If there is any doubt that the emotional part of the brain is connected to the gut, just look at the terminology surrounding the gastrointestinal system. There are gut feelings, gut instincts, gut reactions. If we are brave, we are gutsy; if not, we are gutless. This language is visceral and organ-related. The GI tract is responsive to many human situations. The stomach is one of the most responsive organs in the body, reacting in its spasms and emptying and contractions to almost every emotion and sensation. This mind-gut connection is not simply metaphorical; our brain and our gut are connected by an extensive network of neurons, hormones and chemicals that constantly travel back and forth in a bidirectional fashion.

The Second Brain

In the early 90's, Michael Gershon at Columbia University wrote a book entitled "The Second Brain". He was referring to the nerve cells in the GI tract that act as a distinct brain which can control gut functions all by itself. He called it the enteric nervous system (ENS). It is really the "first brain" since it existed for millions of years before the arrival of the big brain.

The Bugs

Bugs have been our constant companions throughout our evolution. There are about 100 trillion microorganisms in the gut from over 40,000 species and 100 times the number of genes in the human genome. This amounts to about 2 1/2 pounds of bugs, mostly bacteria, the same weight as the human brain! They are called commensals, from the Latin "eating together". In a commensal relationship, one species benefits while the other is neither harmed nor helped. However, it is more of a mutualistic relationship since both parties' benefit. The microbes have coevolved with host organisms, becoming co-dependent for survival. In a way, we grew up together; there was never a time that mammals existed without microbes. During fetal development, the initial colonization of our microbiome coincides with the development of our nervous system.

Gut to Brain Signaling

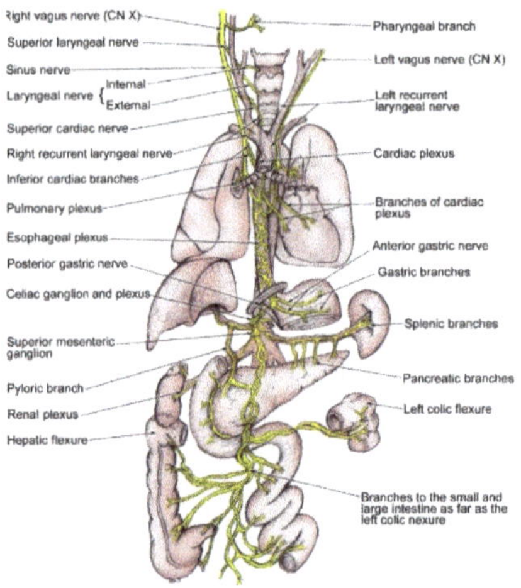

There are multiple mechanisms by which the gut communicates with the brain, via nerves, via a host of signaling molecules produced in the gut wall. The Vagus nerve, the "wanderer", the largest nerve in the body, carries these signals to the brain.

There is a continuous stream of signals from the gut to the brain, but only a small portion of information is consciously perceived, usually that which requires a conscious behavior, such as eating or defecating. Perhaps all of these subconscious signals are what contribute to the mysterious "gut feeling" which is independent of inductive or deductive reasoning.

Brain to Gut Signaling

The brain communicates with the gut through multiple pathways, including the hypothalamic, pituitary, adrenal axis, HPAA, and the autonomic nervous system, ANS. The two key brain structures are the amygdala and the hypothalamus. They receive inputs from multiple brain areas that are constantly monitoring body states, hunger, pain, and food intake. Outputs from the amygdala and hypothalamus via the HPAA and the ANS are referred to as the emotional motor systems, EMS.

The brain can also exert a powerful influence on gut bacteria. Many studies have shown that even mild stress can tip the microbial balance in the gut, making the host more vulnerable to infectious diseases.

The Irritable Bowel Syndrome

Disturbances in the brain-gut axis have been implicated in several chronic disorders, especially the "functional GI disorders" (FGIDs). IBS, irritable bowel syndrome, is the most common of the FGIDs. It can be defined as the presence of recurrent abdominal pain or discomfort in association with a change in bowel habit. IBS accounts for 20-30% of the GI specialists' workload. Like all other MUDs, it has a chronic relapsing course. Similarly, the IBS sufferer most likely also suffers from co-existent mood disorders and anxiety, compared to healthy controls and reports a low quality of life.

Patients with IBS demonstrate increased sensitivity to balloon distention of the GI tract, analogous to the pain hypersensitivity of fibromyalgia. The brain has a critical role to play in the generation of maintenance of IBS symptoms. Stressful and traumatic events during early life increase the chance of developing IBS, and stress in adult life plays a crucial role during the first onset and symptom flare. *In an earlier chapter, we examined the effect of maternal separation on rat pups and how early-life stress led to an amplified pain response with colonic distention. What was even more remarkable, however, than observing the consistent effects of maternal separation were the insights into the biological mechanisms underlying these behavioral changes. Whole-brain circuits and connections develop differently in the separated pups. The neglected stressed animals had greater production of the critical stress molecule, corticotropin-releasing factor (CRF). The amygdala increased in size and density, and the normal circuits (hippocampal/cortical), which regulate the stress response, became less efficient, the perfect formula for a pain response disproportionate to the initiating stimuli. (But what is also remarkable and hopeful for the future is the observations of Gosselin. In a 2010 paper in Gastroenterology, researchers showed that riluzole reverses visceral sensitivity in stressed-out rats. Could it be in the future that a medication may reverse the effects of childhood trauma?)*

Unfortunately, clinicians do not consistently inquire about or address the impact of early life events on their patients' health and symptom profile. In a 1990 study on the impact of sexual and physical abuse in women with functional or organic GI disorders, only 17% of providers knew of their patients' abuse history. GI specialists, like all doctors, obey the dictum, "when the only tool you have is a hammer, every problem looks like a nail". In the case of the gastroenterologist the "hammer" is the endoscope, from the top and from the bottom, quick and profitable. Who has the time to listen to bellyaching?

It is important to point out that not all patients with IBS and other medically mysterious disorders are victims of abuse or neglect. Social learning plays a role in other MUDs. Illness behavior occurs when parents increase attention to their children's abdominal complaints, or parents with IBS behave in a manner that demonstrates a preoccupation and obsession with their illness. Alterations in brain anatomy are not the only, nor the primary, factors involved in the development of IBS and other medically unexplained disorders.

In 2005, Barry Marshall and Robin Warren were awarded the Nobel Prize in physiology for the discovery of H. pylori and its association with peptic ulcer, long thought to be a psychosomatic disorder. Physicians and scientists who adhere to the pain = injury model felt vindicated. For them, "organicity" is the key to respectability, but this is not an either-or proposition. Estimates suggest that approximately 60-80 % of individuals with H. pylori may not show any symptoms and 10% of patients with proven peptic ulcer are not infected with H. pylori. In this disorder, as in all others, the challenge is to determine the relative contribution of nature in the form of genetics and physiology and nurture in the form of upbringing, environment and other influences.

Michael Gershon: The Second Brain. Harper Perennial. 1998
Emeran Mayer: The Mind-Gut Connection. Harper Collins. 2016
O'Moloney: "Early Life Stress Induces Visceral Hypersensitivity in Mice. Neuroscience Letters. Oct. 2011
O'Mahoney, et. al. "Early Life Adversity in Brain Development". Neuroscience 2015.
Prusator, D.K.: "Neurobiology of Early Life Stress and Visceral Pain". Neurogastroenterology Model (2016) 28, 1290-1305
Drossman, D.A.: Sexual and Physical Abuse in Women With Functional or Organic Gastrointestinal Disorders. Amer. Int. Med. 1990, 113-33
Gosselin, et.al., "Riluzole Normalizes Early-Life Stress-Induced Visceral Hypersensitivity in Rats." Gastroenterology 2010; 138: 2418-2425.

Chapter 22

Back Pain

Back pain is probably the most common pain complaint across the globe and is the single leading cause of disability worldwide. 60 million Americans suffer from chronic low back pain. Nonspecific low back pain is the most common presentation, with 90% of cases having no clear causation. It is more prevalent in women. It is also the fourth most expensive condition for employers in the US.

We are the most successful primate on the planet, but we pay a price. We were never meant to stand upright, although that did confer enormous advantages, enabling us to better see prey or enemy, but it came with a price. When humans stood upright, they took a spine that had evolved for climbing and moving in trees and rotated it 90° so it was vertical. But then, so as not to obstruct the birth canal and to get the torso balanced above our feet, the spine has to curve inwards, creating the hollow of our back, lordosis. This is why our spines are shaped like an S. Becoming bipedal has placed severe biomechanical stress on the lower vertebrae, leading to back pain.

At about 20 years of age, disc degeneration begins, and the space between the vertebrae shrinks. Over time, this leads to the growth of new bone, which can impinge on nerve roots, causing pain. Almost everybody over the age of 30 has some form of abnormality on their MRI scan. Lumbar spinal stenosis (stenosis means "narrowing") is a very common clinical syndrome among adults over the age of 65, with increasing prevalence because of an aging population.

Nonspecific low back pain, "lumbago" is the most common presentation with no clear-cut pathology. This accounts for about 90% of cases of low back pain. The pain originates from mechanical and chemical irritation of pain receptors in the lumbar spinal segments, an inevitable consequence of aging, but as the condition persists, psychological and social factors inevitably lead to the chronic state, where it truly becomes a medically unexplained disorder.

Back pain does not always follow the pain equals injury model. Up to 60% of patients presenting to outpatient spinal centers suffer from depression and anxiety. Living with chronic pain can certainly lead to depression, but careful long-term studies show that depression precedes the development of chronic low back pain. In a prospective study of 9909 adults without pre-existing low back pain, individuals with depression were nearly three times as likely to develop chronic low back pain over a 2-year period.

Psychosocial risk factors were much more powerful in predicting low back pain disability than structural abnormalities. The overuse of opioid pain medications has also contributed to the epidemic of low back pain. The prolonged use of opioid medications has a paradoxical effect; it leads to a heightened pain perception, opioid-induced hyperalgesia. *It is an unfortunate product of the medical model that all of these factors are largely ignored when it comes to treatment.*

Treatment

The "three epidural steroid injections" are enshrined as the mainstay of treatment for back pain, but their efficacy is far from clear. Cochrane reviews, which critically evaluate randomized controlled trials (RCTs), found that epidural steroid injections (ESIs) are *probably slightly* more effective than placebo. Many studies show that they can be modestly more effective than placebo for short-term relief of sciatica and radicular pain, but their benefits beyond a few months are minimal or absent. There is much debate on this issue, but Cochrane reviews are unbiased and considered authoritative.

Equally controversial is the use of spinal implantable devices for chronic low back pain. A Cochrane review concluded that spinal cord stimulation (SCS) is no better than placebo for treating low back pain and comes with considerable risks.

Surgery

Laminectomy and spinal fusion procedures have dramatically increased during the last few decades in the US. Spinal surgeries are performed in the US at a rate five times higher than in any other developed country, even though spinal disease and injury are no more prevalent in the US than elsewhere. Little wonder that the direct cost in the US of low back pain has been estimated to be between $12 and $90 billion annually. When compared with other chronic health conditions such as angina and diabetes, low back pain was determined to be the 4th most expensive condition for employers in the United States.

There is a high rate of failure in back surgery procedures. In 2002, there were over one million back surgeries performed in the US. 40-70% have residual back pain. This is not because of poor surgical skills; it is the failure to identify and treat underlying behavioral issues. Patients with psychiatric disorders have worse outcomes and higher risk of developing post-surgical complications.

There are many other reasons why surgery might not be successful, obesity, smoking, opioid dependence, etc., but addressing the "psych" issues could make a substantial difference in outcomes. Prescreening patients before surgery could be invaluable in uncovering depression, anxiety, and history of abuse. Treating these conditions could have a major impact on surgical outcomes. In a study of 27 patients undergoing anterior cervical discectomy and fusion, (ACDF), there were significant improvements in post-op neck pain at one year in patients who received treatment for their anxiety compared with those who had not.

In a study performed by Dr. Jerome Schofferman at the University of California, San Francisco, reported in the journal Spine in 1992, 100 adults with MRI-proven severe lumbar disc disease were interviewed preoperatively for the following:

- physical abuse,
- sexual abuse,
- emotional neglect and abandonment in childhood.
- Loss of one or both parents through divorce or death, and
- drug use at home, either alcohol or prescription drugs.

Patients were assigned to three different groups, none of those risk factors, one or two risk factors, and three or more. All other parameters were strictly regulated to eliminate as much variation as possible. The results were as follows:

- If there were zero risk factors, there was a ninety-five percent chance of success.
- If there were one or two, there was a seventy-five percent chance of success.
- If there were three or more, chances of success were fifteen percent.

Nobody "sacrificed" these patients to look at their brain, but we can rightly assume that the stress factors cited in this study caused changes in the pain circuitry, leading to altered pain perception. There have been many more studies since then that have linked the presence of preexisting comorbid psychiatric conditions to increased health risks, poor treatment outcomes and higher use of healthcare resources. Unfortunately, these studies have had little impact on the treatment of back pain and other forms of chronic pain.

Let me offer a rather facile analogy. When your Tesla, or any other electric vehicle of your choice, malfunctions, you bring it to your local mechanic who is trained in internal combustion technology. He cannot find anything wrong. He is baffled because the problem resides in the computer, the central computing unit, the CPU. Doctors need to start considering our own CPU, THE BRAIN!

Dr. John Sarno, a professor of rehabilitation medicine at New York University School of Medicine, felt that back pain was a psychological disorder. His theory, simply stated, is that back pain develops as a way of unconsciously shifting attention away from uncomfortable feelings such as anger and anxiety. With rare exceptions, Dr. Sarno believed back pain had no structural basis. His work emphasized the importance of the mind in health and has been of enormous benefit to patients worldwide. However, he took his ideas to an extreme degree, attributing too much power to psychological factors. He was all psyche and no soma! His last books promised near miracles, losing touch with reality, thereby reducing the power of his original insights.

One has to be cautious about delving into "mind-body" interactions when treating chronic pain patients. It would not garner you a favorable Yelp review were you to tell a patient with 30 years of chronic low back pain, who wants a refill of their hydrocodone, that their symptoms are "a response to stored trauma and an overflow of repressed emotions." The wise physician introduces such concepts with caution!

P. Polatin: Psych Disorders in Back Pain. Spine. 1993; 18:66-71

Block, A.: The Use of Presurgical Psych Screening to Predict Outcome of Spine Surgery. Spine Journal Vol. 1, Issue 4, July-Aug. 2001. p. 274-282

M. Menendez: Psychiatric Disorders and Major Spine Surgery. Spine Vol. 39, #2, E111-E122

J. Schofferman. Spine Vol. 17, 1992

Chapter 23
Other Central Pain Disorders

The following conditions have little to do with behavioral issues, but are included to highlight the fact that these terrible afflictions are due to changes within the brain and spinal cord, in the CPU. They are examples of the most unbearable pain disorder of all, nerve pain, or "neuropathic" pain

Post-Herpetic Neuralgia

Steven is a 69-year-old gentleman, an engineer by training, who presents with agonizing pain along a portion of the left chest wall. Months before, he had classic shingles. The lesions are gone but the pain persists. He has a marked sensitivity to any form of touch over the affected area. He has rigged up a contraption that prevents any garment from touching the affected area. Gabapentin is the only medication that offers relief.

In pain clinics across the world, neuropathic or nerve pain is the most feared. Neuropathic pain is the type of pain that arises from damage or dysfunction of the nervous system itself, including the peripheral nerves, spinal cord and brain. Damage to the peripheral nerve is the most common, as seen in diabetic neuropathy, post-herpetic neuralgia (the pain that persists after an attack of shingles), or the persistent "sciatica" that persists even after successful surgery.

Nerve pain has very distinctive qualities, including a sense of heat or burning in the affected area. There may be sudden electric shock-like sensations as well as tingling and pins and needles. There is also an increase in sensitivity to painful stimuli and even non-painful stimuli. This phenomenon, called *allodynia*, leads to a state of hypersensitivity wherein even light touch in the affected area is deeply unpleasant. The key to understanding this kind of pain is known as "sensitization", referenced in a previous chapter. It is the process by which pain pathways are rendered more sensitive to any stimuli, even normal touch. The alarm system itself is malfunctioning.

These pain disorders present an enormous challenge, and we have a very limited armamentarium to offer our patients, including antidepressant medication and anti-seizure drugs. Unlike "normal" pain, opioid drugs have little effect.

Thalamic Pain Syndrome

Francesco is a 54-year-old civil engineer with atrial fibrillation. Three years ago, he had a small stroke in the region of the brain called the thalamus. (The thalamus acts as a relay station for all incoming sensory stimuli, except for smell, before they reach the cortex, where the brain processes the various sensations). Three years after the stroke, he is disabled because of the persistent burning pain along the left side of his body. He is taking an antidepressant daily and gabapentin, but they are having minimal impact on his pain.

Typically, this pain is described as burning, aching, or tingling and can be severe and debilitating. The pain typically appears on the opposite side of the body from where the brain damage occurs. If the stroke affects the right thalamus, then the left side of the body may experience the pain. As in the case of every neuropathic pain, treatment can be challenging and frustrating. The mechanism of this type of pain disorder is as mysterious as it is painful.

Phantom Limb Pain

"There's pain where I am and pain where I ain't."
— Moby-Dick, by Herman Melville

Brandon is a 31-year-old man who underwent surgical removal of his entire right leg as a life-saving measure for invasive muscle cancer. He has daily pain of varying intensity in the absent limb, but states that sometimes the itch is worse than the pain. He desperately wants to scratch and often reaches down to scratch the absent limb.

He has tried all the conventional medications and has had a stimulator placed in his spine, which has not been successful. He depends on marijuana and alcohol as his main treatment. He never complains, but I dread his visits. He is a constant reminder of our inability to treat this type of pain.

About 90% of amputees have a phantom sensation at least temporarily, and, in some patients, it may last for years. The feelings of joint rotation, touch, pain, cold and heat all remain. Phantom limb pain is a direct contradiction of the pain = injury model. The commonly accepted explanation for phantom limb is that, though the limb itself is gone, the brain's internal model of it is still present.

Is his pain real? You would be wise not to ask that question in front of this unfortunate man suffering from this bizarre, agonizing disorder. These pain disorders should bury the simplistic pain = injury model.

Trigeminal Neuralgia

"It's a kind of Tic-Dolly-row, they say—worse nor a toothache. Well, well; I don't know what it is, but the Lord keep me from catching it." — Moby-Dick, by Herman Melville

Tic-Dolly-row, tic douloureux, otherwise known as trigeminal neuralgia, TN, is a condition often described as one of the most painful pathologies known to humanity. Prior to effective treatments, it was referred to as the "suicide pain." Thankfully, we now have very effective remedies, including drugs and surgery, which have eliminated the terror associated with this malady.

It is yet another example of a defective alarm system. The alarm bell is ringing, not because of external danger, but because of a defect in the alarm system itself. The precise cause is yet to be identified, but it may be due to compression of the trigeminal nerve that supplies sensation to the face. Whatever the precise pathology, this large sensory nerve becomes hyper-reactive and fires at random or in response to the most trivial stimulus, such as a light touch to the "trigger zone" or brushing one's teeth. It is commonly misdiagnosed since the pain is often localized to a specific tooth, resulting in several dental procedures before the diagnosis is made.

Chapter 24

Hysteria in the Modern Age

From Paralysis to Fatigue and Pain

"Every age has its signature afflictions"
— Byung-Chul Han, philosopher.

Historian of medicine, Edward Shorter, is the author of a fascinating book on the history of psychosomatic disorders entitled *From Paralysis to Fatigue*. In it, he asserts that hysteria has not disappeared but has morphed "from paralysis into fatigue and pain." Shorter maintains that the basic mechanism of hysterical conversion (the expression of emotion and anxiety through physical form) has existed with the same relative frequency across time and cultures. He coined the term "symptom pool" to signify which manifestations of hysteria are acceptable at any given time and which are socially sanctioned. The exotic manifestations of the 19th century have given way to fatigue and pain. With the advent of CT and MRI scanning, it is easy to disprove hysterical paralysis, but it is impossible to disprove fatigue and pain. Elaine Showalter and other feminist writers argue that the manifestations of hysteria are culturally determined and a reaction to the subservient role of women in a patriarchal society.

There have always been fashionable diagnoses. In the early 20th century, a "miracle cure" was advertised by Rexall Pharmaceutical Company to treat "the peculiar exhausted nervous conditions resulting from the continuous rush and tension under which Americans live." The condition? *Americanitis*!

In the 1980s, there was a surge of interest in what was then described as "burnout." Newspapers and magazines offered guidance on how to recognize and manage this condition, and Christina Maslach, a social psychologist at the University of California, Berkeley, developed one of the field's most widely used assessment tools, the Maslach Burnout Inventory (MBI). Over time, the language surrounding these experiences evolved. Terms such as "yuppie flu" emerged in popular discourse, reflecting, in part, shifting cultural attitudes, before giving way to more formalized medical labels.

Conditions such as Chronic Epstein-Barr and Reactive Hypoglycemia gained attention in succession, followed by Chronic Fatigue Syndrome (CFS), also known as Myalgic Encephalomyelitis (ME) or Systemic Exertion Intolerance Disease (SEID), and later Fibromyalgia. The Mayo Clinic defines CFS as "a complicated disorder characterized by extreme fatigue that can't be explained by any underlying condition." More recently, conditions such as Chronic Lyme disease, Long COVID, brain fog, POTS, and CRPS have entered the conversation, further expanding the landscape of medically unexplained disorders.

However, no matter how we label these disorders, as they shape-shift from one era to another, they teach us crucial lessons:

- Human beings have the flexibility in their nervous systems to convert emotions into physical symptoms. Regardless of the ever-changing symptomatology, this is the fundamental process in most medically unexplained disorders.
- Women patients outnumber men in virtually every category of unexplained illness. Feminist historians and critics have rightly emphasized that hysteria was, in part, a response to social conditions that particularly oppressed and constricted women, a sociocultural corset. In a male-dominated society, females repress anger and hostility and convert it to culturally approved symptoms.
- It is important to note that men are not immune to conversion disorders, but one cannot call it hysteria for obvious reasons. After the First World War, there was an epidemic of "shell shock," with a variety of symptoms, including hysterical paralysis, blindness, and bizarre movement disorders.

- Hysteria has not disappeared. It is a foolhardy doctor who would dare utter that word in public, but privately, doctors still talk of hysterical tendencies and hysterical patients.

Every culture has its own unique symptom pool. Koro (Southeast Asia) involves the intense fear that one's genitals are retracting into the body, which can lead to significant anxiety and distress. It is often reported in cultures where traditional beliefs about bodily functions and sexuality are prevalent. Zar (North Africa and the Middle East) involves possession by spirits, leading to symptoms such as dissociation, altered consciousness, and physical complaints. Susto (Latin America) refers to a condition believed to result from a traumatic event, causing a person's soul to be lost. Symptoms include physical ailments like muscle pains and diarrhea, as well as psychological distress. Amok (Southeast Asia) refers to a specific behavioral phenomenon characterized by sudden, intense episodes of uncontrolled rage or violence. It is often seen as a reaction to extreme stress, humiliation, or personal crisis. In the West, we also "run amok" and have nervous breakdowns, but without the attendant violence.

Our symptom pool has no such drama. Our MUDs are subjective and internal in nature, with no external signs to communicate distress. They are often ridiculed and dismissed by medical doctors, often with the comment, "just a female problem." (Since most of the sufferers are female.) Medicine must undergo a radical shift to accommodate these disorders and reclaim them from the charlatans who exploit them for profit.

The first step in reclaiming these disorders is to establish their real brain disorders, based on alterations in brain structure and function. Psychology, behavior, culture, and social factors will always play a role, but it is the brain that processes these factors and ultimately determines the response.

However we categorize these conditions, they have always been with us. The presentations may change with time, but no physician, past or present, has been exempt from dealing with these disorders.

For thousands of years, they have been a source of puzzlement and frustration. (I confess that a clear-cut, obvious disease is sometimes a relief!)

However, as always in dealing with human beings, there is a dark side. Not every medically unexplained disorder is the result of childhood stress or deep-rooted psychological factors. There is no doubt that "secondary gain" plays a huge role. Secondary gain refers to the additional advantages or benefits that a person may receive from their condition or behavior, particularly in the context of illness or psychological issues. These gains may include receiving sympathy and attention from family and friends, avoidance of responsibilities and, of course, financial benefits. There can be obvious financial benefits to being sick. In one of the first editions of a magazine devoted to fibromyalgia called "Fibromyalgia Aware", 60% of the articles were devoted to receiving disability benefits. This type of manipulation confronts physicians frequently and it is easy to become cynical. However, one must beware of throwing the baby out with the bathwater.

Edward Shorter: From Paralysis to Fatigue. The Free Press, 1993

Chapter 25

"What is to be done"? —V. I. Lenin (1902)

Any attempt to change the medical model or the medical culture faces extraordinary difficulties. Physicians, insurance carriers and the patient population are all firmly wedded to that traditional medical model. We cannot expect any assistance from the psychiatric professions, who are mired in their own sea of confusion. As the head of the APA, Leon Eisenberg, once stated, "Once upon a time, psychiatry was brainless; now it's mindless" (Leon Eisenberg). With the virtual collapse of the 19th century Freudian model, psychiatry has swung to biologism, but that has not succeeded very well. They are confronted with the same problem that Freud experienced when he tried for a biological psychology. There is simply not enough neuroscience. But that has not discouraged the National Institute of Mental Health, NIMH, which has advocated taking the "mental" out of the equation. "Mental disorders are disorders of the brain". (Oct 14, 2018). Now that's biologism!

George Engel and The Biopsychosocial Model

There have been several attempts in the past to reconcile mind and body, psyche and soma, psychology and biology.

In 1922, Felix Deutsch introduced the term "psychosomatic" into medical literature. In 1939, the first issue of the "Journal of Psychosomatic Medicine" was published, and finally, in 1982, the word psychosomatic appeared in the Oxford English Dictionary. The most prominent figure in the attempt to revamp the medical model was George Engel, 1913-1999.

Trained as an internist and psychiatrist, he was instrumental in developing and teaching psychosomatic medicine at the University of Rochester in Rochester, NY. He realized that the medical model of disease was no longer adequate to address patients' needs. He developed the Biopsychosocial Model, BPSM. It viewed health and illness as the result of interactions between biological, psychological, and social factors. It challenged the biomedical approach, which focuses exclusively on the biological. His paper, published in Science in April 1977, challenged the medical establishment, and the establishment fought back! His colleagues and contemporaries offered the following comments:

"Medicine should concentrate on real diseases and not get lost in the psycho-sociological underbrush. The physician should not be saddled with problems that have arisen from the abdication of the theologian and the philosopher."

Another advocated *a "disentanglement of the organic elements of disease from the psychosocial elements of human malfunction and medicine should deal only with the former."* (Good luck with that!)

And finally, the unkindest cut of all, *"the biopsychosocial model is a disingenuous euphemism for psychosomatic illness."* (which of course is imaginary and "mental")

The biopsychosocial model is now a historical footnote, but it was a well-meaning attempt to bridge the chasm between mind and body. The critics who gleefully pointed out its deficiencies have not yet come up with anything better. Like it or not, physicians have to deal with the underbrush. Any doctor who wishes to avoid it should consider a career in veterinary medicine. Any attempt to shift the paradigm, to develop a more inclusive medical model, faces a monolithic challenge. However, refusing to be discouraged, I offer my "Notes from the Underbrush".

Engel, G.: The Need for a New Medical Model. Science. 1977; 196:129-136
S. Nassir Ghaemi. The Rise and Fall of the Biopsychosocial Model. John Hopkins. 2010.

Chapter 26

"A Modest Proposal" — Jonathan Swift (1729)

"To every complicated problem there is a simple solution and it's usually wrong."
— H. L. Mencken

"Unless our academic medical centers broaden the base of their activities and interests to give psychological elements as much continuing attention as is now given biologic aspects, medicine's crisis and public disappointment and chagrin will continue and deepen."
— Irving Lewis, The Sick Citadel (1983)

The Training of the Physician.

1. Mind- Brain-Body curriculum

Imagine if you told physicians in training that 70% of the disorders they will encounter in their professional life will not feature in their curriculum? They would think you were insane, but such is the case. The medical student must always be grounded in the traditional medical model, and that will always be an essential part of the training, but there must be an acknowledgment of the role of stress, behavior and culture in the causes of disease and "unease". The medically unexplained disorders, the 70%, deserve to be acknowledged as a major cause of human suffering and can no longer be ignored. Gray's Anatomy (the book, not the TV series) will always be the foundation of medical education, but much more is needed.

Every medical student should be exposed to patients with mood and behavioral disorders. The chasm between medicine and "psych" should be bridged early in their training. There should be a mandatory 6-12-week course dealing with mind-brain-body disorders: Not esoteric philosophy but elegant neuroscience. There are many brilliant thinkers writing about the interplay between mind, brain, and body, but they might as well be writing in Sanskrit, so meager is their influence on medical training. The works of Robert Sapolsky, Bruce McEwen, Joseph LeDoux, Michael Meaney and others should be an intrinsic part of the curriculum. The neurobiology of stress is the most important subject in bridging the gap between psyche and soma and they are pioneers in understanding how stress impacts the brain and body. Their insights reveal the intimate brain-body connection and enable the physician to talk about brain-body disorders rather than "mental" ones. The doctor should be able to explain how stress, either past or present, alters brain structure and function, validating the patient's complaints, giving legitimacy to both patient and doctor. The goal is not to produce physician/philosophers, but at least the young doctor must appreciate that human beings are more than a collection of organs wrapped in a bag of skin.

2. Females also have bodies and brains

Sex, Biology. There must be a part of medical education devoted to the unique needs of the female patient, involving sex (biology) and gender (culture). Little, if any, distinction is made between the psychophysiology of the male and female. The female body has been largely ignored in clinical trials over the last century. Females are born into a patriarchal culture that imposes unique stresses in addition to the challenges of an ever-changing hormonal environment. The neuroendocrinology of pregnancy, the postpartum and menopause are largely ignored, even by gynecologists.

Erin is a 47-year-old female, entering menopause. She feels she is losing her mind, that her ability to function in an executive role in a global company is compromised. Her moods are erratic, with jagged spikes of suicidal depression that were unknown to her. These changes are even more worrisome than the wretched hot flashes that can happen at any time, day or night. She sought the help of a gynecologist to see if hormone replacement therapy might help. She was advised to consider "axe-throwing" as a way of relieving tension.

Gender, Culture. Physicians should also be educated in the gender (cultural) issues which are relevant in female distress. In a patriarchal society, females are often victims of abuse and discrimination and are trained to internalize their feelings. An in-depth study of feminist literature is hardly necessary, but physicians should have some awareness of the impact of culture and societal values in the expression of disease and unease in females. If the vast majority of those suffering from the mysterious medical disorders are female, then we had better get to know them!

3. The patient interview: How to listen

Listening has become a lost art. The most important part of being a healer is to listen, empathize, and validate. You cannot do that if you are tapping on your tablet or computer. A frequent complaint is, "they never even looked at me". I know that time is limited, but it doesn't take much to turn to your patient and say, "Tell me a little about yourself." Those few minutes may tell you a great deal about the person, often more than MRIs and CTs. The words of Sir William Osler should be written in stone: "A good doctor treats disease, a great doctor treats the person who has the disease". A busy family doctor with 30 patients sniffling and coughing in the waiting room doesn't have much time for listening, but for those in specialty care, those minutes of active listening can reveal more than the multiple imaging studies.

It is important to inquire about early childhood and adolescent abuse when appropriate. Many patients sequester traumatic memories as though the past has no bearing on their current distress. It is a delicate process to extract a history of abuse, especially sexual abuse in childhood but it is worthwhile. I am often asked, "Why bother to unearth these childhood traumas, when there's nothing you can do about it?" Shakespeare's Macbeth asked the same plaintive question to his lady's doctor:

"Canst thou not minister to a mind diseased,

pluck from the memory a rooted sorrow,

raze out the written troubles of the brain

and with some sweet oblivious antidote

cleanse the stuffed bosom of that perilous stuff

which weighs upon the heart?"

I am not as fatalistic as the doctor who replied, "therein the patient must minister to himself".

One cannot undo the past, but it is a very healing process for patients to make the connection between events of the past and their current symptoms. The pain circuitry in the brain is actually altered by stress, especially in childhood. Relating symptoms to actual brain changes is validating, removing the stigma of "it's all in your mind." Time and time again, patients have reported that being validated, understanding the link between early childhood stress and changes within the brain, has been the first step in the healing process. Validation and empathy are powerful medicines

Chapter 27

From Bench to Bedside. Translating Brain-body Medicine to the Clinic

Integrating mind-brain-body medicine into mainstream Healthcare is an enormous challenge. The Cartesian mind-body split still dominates the landscape for physicians, patients, and insurance companies alike. There is a profusion of emerging disciplines attempting to fuse mind, brain, and body into a coherent approach. These include neurogastroenterology, neuroendocrinology, neuroimmunology, neurocardiology, neurogynecology, neurourology, psycho-neuroendocrinology, psychoneuroimmunology and integrative medicine. The psychiatric field is also attempting the crossover approach with neuropsychiatry, biological psychiatry, neuropsychology, and interpersonal neurobiology. These are all very welcome additions, but the cumbersome neologisms merely emphasize how fragmented we still are. I believe the term ***neurobehavioral medicine*** is the simplest and most embracing term of all. It embraces all of the above-mentioned hybrid specialties, although there may be a different "target organ." It also brings psychiatric disorders into the fold; these are brain disorders, not "mental" illness. (We should avoid the term *neuropsychiatry* for obvious reasons!)

Neurobehavioral Medicine in the Clinic: Needless to say, the proper selection of patients is paramount. A fractured tibia does not need brain-body medicine. The patient with an acute disc herniation in the lumbosacral spine doesn't need a psychotherapist. (In fact, here is a situation where a well-placed epidural injection could have real value.) The more chronic the disorder, the less likely there is a magic bullet. In these disorders, healing is a process, not an event. The medical culture is still doctor-centric, but no individual physician can handle complex neurobehavioral disorders. It takes a team.

Corrine is a 36-year-old attorney who developed a sudden onset of left-sided weakness and numbness approximately 6 months prior. There appeared to be no precipitating factors, and every conceivable test has proven negative. She has been diagnosed with migraine-related stroke, even though there is no evidence of stroke, and she has never had a migraine attack! Her examination, with "give-way weakness" and non-anatomical sensory loss, confirms that this is a functional neurologic disorder, FND.

Helping this woman demands an interdisciplinary approach. The physical therapist gently encourages ever-increasing mobility on the affected left side; the cognitive behavioral therapist will gently probe the origins of the disorder and, with time, will help the patient to reframe the meaning of her symptoms and explore precipitating causes. This is done slowly while also teaching meditation and relaxation techniques which are held in group sessions. The role of the MD is peripheral, but it is important they validate the reality of the condition and emphasize that it is "organic", but happily a reversible condition unlike stroke or tumor. They will explain how stress affects brain structure and function, and how psychology affects biology.

Psychiatric disorders will be viewed as neurobehavioral disorders treated in an interdisciplinary fashion. In addition to conventional psychiatric medications, there will be special emphasis on other available treatments such as transcranial magnetic stimulation, especially the Stanford accelerated format of transcranial magnetic stimulation, SAINT (Stanford Accelerated Intelligent Neuromodulation Therapy), which accomplishes results in a much more compressed timeframe. The use of intranasal ketamine has proven to be of value in *treatment-resistant depression, and in the coming months (years?),* we may expect FDA approval for the use of psychedelic compounds to treat intractable depression, OCD, ADHD, and other neurobehavioral disorders. There is a great deal of optimism surrounding these compounds, which offer a more direct and immediate pathway to recovery. We may be approaching the "Ozempic Era" in psychiatry, but much work has to be done before these medicines become mainstream.

Psychological services are an essential part of the clinic, with cognitive-behavioral therapy appearing to be the most appropriate in this setting. Since stress is at the core of many neurobehavioral disorders, a stress management program is an essential component. A stress management program would be of great value for anxiety, fatigue, gastrointestinal symptoms, insomnia, depression, sleep disorder, chronic pain, headaches and especially for medically unexplained disorders. Many patients with these disorders have an overactive sympathetic nervous system, always in a fight or flight mode with all the subsequent physiologic accompaniments such as increased heart rate, blood pressure, muscle tension, accompanied by increased levels of cortisol and noradrenaline. The goal of stress management is to induce a parasympathetic state with increased vagal tone. This can be achieved by a wide variety of techniques. The use of meditation and mindfulness has proven to be extremely beneficial. Meditation is no longer a fringe practice associated with exotic gurus; it has entered the mainstream and become a billion-dollar industry.

(There are several successful programs adopting the holistic approach in the United States. A notable example is the Benson-Henry Institute for Mind-Body Medicine at Massachusetts General Hospital. Their "Stress Management and Resiliency Training", SMART, receives referrals from primary care physicians and specialists alike. In a brief publication in the New England Journal of Medicine in 2020, Michelle L Dossett of the Benson-Henry Institute wrote, "belief in these techniques is not necessary to realize benefit. Indeed, randomized controlled trials have suggested improved health outcomes and quality of life in multiple physical and mental health conditions that are related to or exacerbated by stress.)

Brain Health: The neurobehavioral center is not merely focused on disease but on brain health. The field of dementia is an example of how an interdisciplinary approach can lead to successful outcomes with early detection of risk factors and initiation of treatment before the disease progresses. Technology is of paramount importance. Its importance is illustrated by the fact that patients often spend large sums of money on imaging studies such as SPECT (Single-Photon Emission Computed Tomography), which offer pretty, colored pictures and little else. Functional imaging of the brain, fMRI, is still not routinely available, but advanced neuroimaging with specialized MRI techniques is becoming more accurate and is an important part of brain evaluation.

Assembling the Team

An interdisciplinary team may include a neurologist, a psychiatrist, a psychologist, a physical therapist, an acupuncturist, and a biofeedback therapist. But a word of caution.... The idea of a programmatic approach is great in theory, but it will run afoul of the insurance carriers. Many interdisciplinary programs have disappeared because the carrier will carve out components of the program, paying for some and denying others.

The basic personnel required are often present but need to be integrated into the team.

1. A Nurse Navigator, the intake person who gathers the medical records, often very extensive and orients the patient to the program. Initial evaluation will consist of specific computer-driven cognitive tests.
2. A psychologist who will evaluate patients and decide on the most appropriate approach to treatment. There is no data as to the most effective type of psychological intervention, but Cognitive-Behavioral Therapy, CBT, seems to be the most useful in this setting
3. Education, preferably done in a group setting, will explain the link between mind, brain, and body, especially the effects of chronic stress on pain processing.
4. Physical therapy. The focus will be on mobility and flexibility, not passive modalities such as heat, ultrasound and massage. (HUM)!
5. Biofeedback is often very valuable in relaxation therapy. It is often the simplest way of demonstrating the mind-brain-body connectivity.

6. Mindfulness and meditation have proven to be very effective in treating anxiety disorders and pain.
7. Eye Movement Desensitization and Reprocessing (EMDR) can be helpful in achieving rapid results in patients with childhood trauma or PTSD. It is not without controversy, but it is endorsed by the World Health Organization.

Consultants to the Neurobehavioral Center will include a gynecologist to address the female aspects of the patient's symptoms, especially to manage menopausal symptoms and to offer guidance on hormone replacement therapy and postpartum depression. Addiction specialist is crucial since substance abuse disorder, prescribed or otherwise, rarely benefits unless the substance abuse is addressed. Other specialties will be available on demand, including neurosurgery and pain management.

We can expect as much resistance from patients as from physicians when presented with a brain-body approach. Patients entrenched in the model may feel that their symptoms are being devalued and that such a treatment approach is just new-age poppycock! People must be slowly educated in the value of these other therapies, and we must always be realistic in what we can achieve. A 74-year-old patient who has lived with chronic pain for many years and who has relied on opioids and epidural injections will not respond well to the suggestion of mind-body medicine. It will be a slow transformation from the "find it and fix it" model; change will come only if the Brain-Body approach is seen to be a more efficient use of resources. But that will depend on measurement!

Chapter 28

The Measurement Problem

Economics is the major determining factor in many areas of life and especially in health care. If we could put a price tag on the cost of MUDs, which would be staggering, it could initiate change, much more than any philosophizing. But it is impossible to measure the cost of these disorders when we have no idea as to their dimensions. Without the International Classification of Diseases (ICD) codes, they do not exist. There are multiple ICD-10 codes for medically unexplained disorders, but they are laden with the innuendo of mental or psychological (read "imaginary, unreal"). Insurance carriers may deny care for these patients, ("we don't cover psych") and patients are fearful that a "psych" diagnosis may impact on their work status or their ability to qualify for life or disability insurance in the future. We need new diagnoses and ICD codes that are not stigmatizing. Here are a few creative alternatives, courtesy of ChatGPT:

Perception-Related Distress Syndrome (PRDS). "A disorder where individuals experience significant emotional distress stemming from their perception of physical symptoms, without identifiable medical causes". (Not bad, and it has a catchy acronym.)

Emotional Response Syndrome (ERS). "A condition in which emotional states manifest as physical symptoms, affecting daily functioning without any organic pathology". (I would take issue with the concept of "organic")

Adaptive Response Disorder (ARD). "A condition characterized by maladaptive psychological responses to stressors that switch to physical forms, resulting in chronic pain or discomfort." (Great title and acronym, but not the rest)

Stress Sensitivity Disorder (SSD). "A condition where normal stressors lead to exaggerated psychological and physical reactions resulting in chronic discomfort." (Good but would eliminate "psychological")

Sensory Overload Maladaptation Syndrome (SOMS). "A disorder where individuals are hypersensitive to sensory inputs, resulting in psychosomatic responses and discomfort." (Definitely not!)

Perhaps it is time for the American Medical Association, AMA, to enter the 21st century and do what the psychiatrists have been doing for decades, adapt to changing times and values, and develop our own medical Diagnostic and Statistical Manual, DSM, and ICD codes that encompass all varieties of human suffering.

Of course, Artificial Intelligence is playing a much greater role than merely suggesting imaginative terminology names for perplexing mind-brain-body disorders. The mystique of the doctor is being challenged by the availability of data and information that is now available with the push of a button. And not just data. Claude and ChatGPT offer diagnoses and treatment plans that are eerily accurate and prescient. Admittedly, I still chafe a little when a patient tells me, "I have done my research" and then proceeds to upstage me with their diagnosis. (It is especially galling when they are right!)

The aura of the physician still lingers, although somewhat dimmed. It is still a vital ingredient in the healing process. It resides in an "uber" level that transcends data. Perhaps it is wisdom. There is a framework cited in information science, the D-I-K-W pyramid. (Data, information, knowledge, and wisdom). Data, information and knowledge are available to all, but wisdom is a rarer commodity. T.S. Elliot wrote, "Where is the wisdom we have lost in knowledge? Where is the knowledge we have lost in information?" That wisdom part is still elusive to machines, which is why physicians will be around for just a little while longer.

www.ingramcontent.com/pod-product-compliance
Lightning Source LLC
LaVergne TN
LVHW071743071126
851857LV00045B/2072